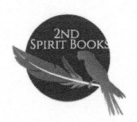

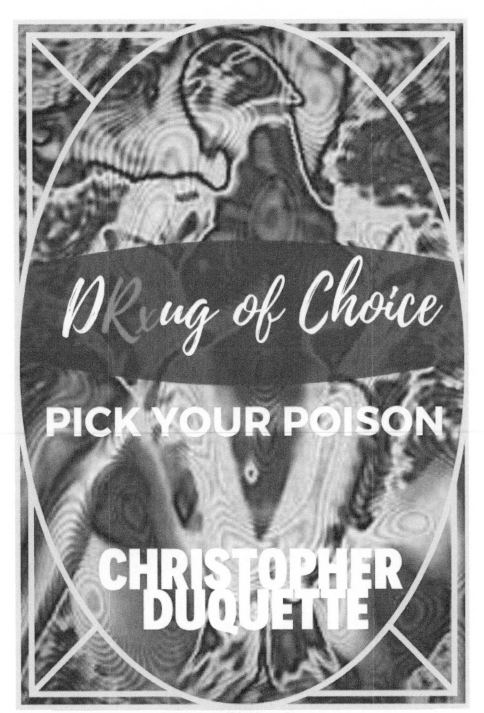

DRxug of Choice

PICK YOUR POISON

CHRISTOPHER DUQUETTE

Published in the United States of America

DonnaInk Publications, L.L.C. | 2nd Spirit Books

DRxug of Choice

PICK YOUR POISON

CHRISTOPHER DUQUETTE

2nd Spirit Books Imprint
Publishers Since 2012
An imprint of DonnaInk Publications, L.L.C.
601 McReynolds Street
Carthage, NC 28327

Library of Congress Cataloging-in-Publication.
Duquette, Christopher, author.
  Title: "DRxug of Choice: Pick Your Poison" / Mr. Christopher Duquette.
    176 p. cm.
      Subjects: BIO031000 - Biography & Autobiography / LGBT; BIO033000 - Biography & Autobiography / Performing Arts see Entertainment & Performing Arts; SOC064000 - Social Science / LGBT Studies / General; SOC064010 - Social Science / LGBT Studies / Bisexual Studies; SOC012000 - Social Science / LGBT Studies / Gay Studies; SOC017000 - Social Science / LGBT Studies / Lesbian Studies; SEL001000 - Self-Help / Addiction; SEL026000 - Self-Help / Substance Abuse & Addictions / General; SEL006000 - Self-Help / Substance Abuse & Addictions / Alcohol; SEL013000 - Self-Help / Substance Abuse & Addictions / Drugs.

Identifiers: ISBN – 13 - 978-1-947704-19-0 (alk. paper) | ISBN – 978-1-947704-24-4 (digital).

Printed in the United States of America
First Edition: 12 11 10 9 8 7 6 5 4 3 2 1; 2019. All Rights Reserved.

For more information contact:
DonnaInk Publications, L.L.C.
601 McReynolds St., Carthage, NC 28327
www.donnaink.com

OTHER WORKS

By Christopher Duquette

Homo Gogo Man: A Fairytale About A Boy Who Grew Up In Discoland

REVIEWS

Of Homo GoGo Man

This book beautifully and tragically chronicles the halcyon days of New York's . . .

This book beautifully and tragically chronicles the halcyon days of New York's dance club culture and the rise and fall of one of its truly glamorous devotees. It's a must read to understand the difficulties and wounds of growing up as a gay man in the 1970's and 80's and the brutal addiction that can sometimes flower from that damage.

~JJ

His Love of Dance & Disco

Hilarious & very entertaining! Adored following Xristo as he discovers NYC, his love of dance & disco, drowning in partying excesses and finding his way back out. A thoroughly amusing and enjoyable ride - highly recommend it!

~Angela Charters

Love this Book!

Quick read ... Author explains the disco era well. Good story that I could easily see as a movie! His journey and discovery of being a gay man in a small town may help someone who is just coming out.

~Carla

Five Stars!

I thought it was an amazing journey to an era of a dance...awesome.

~Storm Bryant

DEDICATION

Respectfully agnostic, I am grateful for three men no longer on this earth who continue to frequent my dreams as well as make themselves accessible to me for support during my waking hours during moments of strife: Christopher, Shary, & my father Jeremiah. I would also like to give an award to gifted photographer and long-term friend Lucien, who documented my zany image in photogenically beautiful photographs that I am proud to display to the world as the boy who grew up with low self-esteem, but incarnated the facade of a star.

To all the women in my life who have loved me without sexting me:

My mother and confidant Jacqueline Duquette, my soulmate sister Sheryl, Aussie Angela who always seemed to need a man in her bed to validate herself until she met her match in matrimony, and my unconventional publisher, Ms. Donna Lee Quesinberry, who recognizes my talent, acknowledged my ambition, has broken the business barrier by allowing me to be her friend in life as well as my champion to release a revised 2nd edition of my virgin publication, *Homo GoGo Man*, and give me the green light to release my creative essence again in this second published book, a work of love, sweat, blood and guts that I only hope finds an audience that takes it earnestly as well as amusing.

And, finally to Storm Orion, for allowing me to fall back into Love, Life, and Him.

TABLE OF CONTENTS

OTHER WORKS.. ix
By Christopher Duquette ix

REVIEWS.. xi
Of Homo GoGo Man xi

DEDICATION xiii

TABLE OF CONTENTS.. xv

FOREWORD xvii
Jump Aboard & Enjoy the Scenery xvii

INTRODUCTION xxi
The Substance Abuse Merry-Go-Round xxi

EPIGRAPH... xxvii

CHAPTER 1 1
Spontaneous Combustion 1

CHAPTER 2 7
Adolescent Revolution.. 7

CHAPTER 3 25
Recovery Culture 25

CHAPTER 4 41
Non-Elective Institutionalization.................................... 41

CHAPTER 5 49
   Highly Medicated Individual 49

CHAPTER 6 65
   One Excruciating Day At A Time...65

CHAPTER 7 81
   Employable RX Addict..81

CHAPTER 8 91
   Black Market Rx a Pill A Day Keeps the Doctors Away.........91

CHAPTER 9 99
   Dr. RxXnX...99

CHAPTER 10... 117
   Acute Xanax Abuse 117

CHAPTER 11 135
   Treatment Advocacy 135

ABOUT THE AUTHOR 145
   Christopher Duquette 145

FOREWORD

Jump Aboard & Enjoy the Scenery

When Mr. Christopher Duquette approached me regarding his title, *"Homo GoGo Man: A Fairytale About A Boy Growing Up in Discoland"* as a new publisher I wasn't hesitant. At the time, uncertain about the specific genres DonnaInk **Publications, L.L.C.** would undertake – Christopher struck me as an individual to work with while getting our proverbial publishing house wings underway.

With a strong faith-based upbringing and personal belief system, I was" educated to be mindful while embracing diversity and in the past year, largely due to Mr. Duquette and his readers, the 2nd Spirit Books Imprint was created and is derived from Native American terminology regarding alternative lifestyles. This was prior to my knowledge of Mr. Duquette's Native American visions and seems even more befitting now . . . it appears greater forces were at work than that of author and publisher.

Throughout our association, Christopher has remained a considerate and ethical individual; while straightforward, much like his writing style, he is never offensive while direct in sharing synopses of life events and we have shared many stories time and again. Chris is also forthright in sharing the facts about prejudices and/or hardships encountered as a homosexual. Events in Mr. Duquette's life have not been due to his reality – rather inflicted on his life and he shares a lot about the human spirit and the understanding we are all our own person with our own testament in our journey toward our own concept of Nirvana.

For this title, 2nd Spirit Books did not perform an exacting editorial. The integrity, imagery and verbiage remain raw. Certainly, heartfelt. While it would be good to be enabled to state Mr. Duquette's experiences are 100% unique – I believe, "DRxug of Choice: Pick Your Poison," is going to resonate, and then validate, readers' experiences from all walks of life. It is good to share this resonance and it is equally saddening there is one, but Chris's story provides the proverbial light at the end of the tunnel and in time to enjoy the scenery. A heartfelt hope for readers to jump aboard Mr. Duquette's recovery train and view the positive lens of shared futurist abundance is levied with the production of this title.

Both *"Homo GoGo Man: A Fairytale About A Boy Growing Up In Discoland,"* and *"DRxug of Choice: Pick Your Poison,"* receive excellent feedback from industry and readers as first-person accounts of real life where staying strong while remaining true to thine own self demonstrates hutzpah folks often don't exude when grappling similar events. No matter your understanding of, or belief regarding, LGBTQ lifestyles, this title shares organic truths all readers will find interesting. The ability to embrace oneself, even in our worst circumstances, is not the easiest undertaking in life and to do so with brevity is even more unusual. Every person on their mission of humanity holds elements from the past where we've righted a wrong, missed a proverbial bullet, gotten through a rough spot, or beheld miracles of living – balancing life events and formulating a life plan – where experiences transition into golden nuggets of comprehension is what we people aspire to achieve.

Additionally, today's marketplace is riddled with awareness regarding the current pharmaceutically induced results of our fast-food medicinal complexities and how excess, at the very least within the American culture has driven addiction and a need for recovery to the forefront of national causes and the daily news. Moving from knowledge to re-creation of one's existence is an evolutionary step not every individual achieves and lives to write about.

Thankfully, for us, Christopher Duquette is a writer who has.

If you haven't experienced addiction and recovery personally, statistics state you know someone who has – hopefully those good souls have all recovered . . . because over 300 million people die annually throughout the world due to alcohol alone. Over 54 million Americans over age 12 misused prescription drugs in 2018. Over 21 million Americans are addicted to alcohol or drugs. 90% of people with addictions began to drink or use drugs before age 18. Heroin use today starts at age 12 and older and in 2018, 1 million heroin addicts shot heroin for the first time. Annually, nearly 2 million people abuse opioids and many of them began using opioids from prescription and suicide is the 10th leading cause of death in the United States of America . . . but isn't all the above slow suicide?

Christopher Duquette shares intimate, sometimes guttural and gross, details about life and learning to live it beyond phobias, paranoia, weaknesses derived from preconceived gauges for success and on your own terms. His ability to move forward and escape demons in a balanced and educated lifestyle remains insightful and worthy of a read and review.

Thank you, Chris, for continuing to be an exceptional human being to work for, with, and to know. Bravo on approaching the topics addressed in both *"Homo GoGo Man: A Fairytale About A Boy Growing Up In Discoland,"* and *"DRxug of Choice: Pick Your Poison."*

Ms. Donna L. Quesinberry
Founder and President - DonnaInk Publications, L.L.C. & 2nd Spirit Books
Founder and CEO - dpInk Ltd. Liability Company
Founder and Partner - Developmental Arts and Community Services
Author, Business Developer and Strategist, Coach, Freelance Consultant,
Ghostwriter, Poet, Public Speaker, Senior Proposal- and Technical-Writer
Mother of Five Adult Children and Grandmother of Eleven

INTRODUCTION

The Substance Abuse Merry-Go-Round

This is my personal journal documenting the myriad of mind-altering substances I enthusiastically consumed and subsequent remedial treatments I willingly submitted to after being clinically diagnosed by the Medical Community as a threat to myself. After an unsuccessful attempt to take my own life, I was branded as a "Ward of the State"; a danger to myself, forever posing a potential crisis to humanity, which qualified this intimate act to fall within the jurisdiction of local law enforcement. Successful suicides are disguised in public obituaries as "succumbed to a long-term illness", which is an ambiguous reference to a mental disorder, substance abuse overdose, or a homicidal attack to one's own person, making one guilty of one's own murder, only respectfully swept under the rug of public stigma for the family's sake with no formal legal proceedings or restitution.

I am now coming to a junction in consciousness to my current exasperating existence. I have been following the protocol of medical professionals for the past 15 years since I desperately tried four ways from Sunday to end my life. I believe some of the professionals have had my best interest at heart, but obeying their suggestions, respected their medicinal prescriptions, and sharing my most intimate uncensored feelings and thoughts on the record at every scheduled appointment with over 100 medical professionals still has not gotten me any closer to the contentment of life on life's terms until I was granted the aid of a daily regime of narcotic anti-anxiety medication;

Xanax, and its weaker cousin Klonopin. I am stuck in a parallel universe from the one I rode independently for 25 years prior to my suicide, when I first experimented and discovered my idiosyncratic disposition to alter my mind with illicit drugs and alcohol before I bottomed out, leaving me at the mercy of EMS, ER, ICU, Neurosurgeons, Psychologists, Social Workers, untrained attendants employed to resuscitate pathetic victims of bad choices, and repair them so that they may become soldiers in the army of recovery. Besides all the salaries and services rendered, there are layers of administrative bureaucracy that inflate the financial overhead, tallying the cost of keeping me alive enormously more than the most extravagant funeral.

But I am alive today, realistically accepting the ups and downs of life, a bit frustrated that I am dependent on a narcotic medication that I have already experienced is hell to live without. It's a love/hate relationship that I thought I would have grown out of, like a tempestuous lover. And I find it ironic living under the scrutiny of the government I always had an innate antagonist attitude towards. Given my rebellious independent spirit, I find myself humbling and compromising my standards to acquire enough divine gratitude to get through each day. But I still am determined to find my own nirvana; not from a 12 step program, not from a pharmaceutical course of therapy, not from a book written by a scientific journalist based on empirical research that makes no difference to the world order, not from a family member, not from a religion, but from within. I can't ever lose confidence that I am ultimately responsible for my recovery, because I am responsible for getting myself into this mess. I must always advocate for myself. If that means accepting that there are comments in my public health record that I am "difficult", I don't take it personally as I know that I can account for every conversation/discussion/conflict with a medical authority where I respect the parameters of behaving and expressing myself appropriately in a professional environment. The fact I am made aware of these character assassinations by colleagues who know me as a unique human being who is educated, articulate, well-read, candid, and a no-nonsense human being bares evidence that even the medical community is not immune to a client firing them for lack of unacceptable results (i.e.: empathy).

I am now learning to advocate for myself to utilize those medical professsionals, scientists, family members, long-term friends as well as new acquaintances, and strangers I serendipitously encounter in my daily existence, my boyfriend who I intimately share my life with, and guardian angels on this earth and beyond to discern those who can see me, hear me and help me figure out who I am, instead of relying on the diagnostic characterization the medical community implemented over 200 years ago. The same stigmatizing methods realized and still employed by the forefathers of psychological theories (think Sigmoid Freud) are still utilized by the stagnant medical, psychological, pharmacology, and rehabilitation services. The original premise classified substance abusers as a threat to the social order of civilization. They are categorized as suffering from a "mental disorder". New scientific research and alternative recovery methods beginning with hallucinogenic experimentation in the 1960's is still not considered "status quo" by the majority of patients and practitioners who appear to resist any change to their trained and certified professions.

I believe everyone has a unique life story that predetermines their outcome. So, I will start at the beginning of what I remember of my 60 years of life that has left me at this moment where I am motivated to pause so that I may solve the puzzle of my human existence. I want off the merry-go-round before it makes me any sicker.

DRxug of Choice

PICK YOUR POISON

CHRISTOPHER DUQUETTE

EPIGRAPH

Disco music in the '70s was just a call to go wild and party and dance with no thought or conscience or regard for tomorrow.

~ Martha Reeves

The opposite of addiction is not sobriety, but human connection.

— Johann Hari

CHAPTER 1

Spontaneous Combustion

I am the quintessential middle child of an attractive family of five, incubated with upper middle-class suburban entitlement in a quant town nestled amid Hudson Valley, New York. My handsome father coupled with his equally genetically gorgeous high school sweetheart, my mother, to become legally married at the shared age of 20, in the year 1956, when matrimony offered more chance of achieving the American Dream, the opportunity of prosperity and success regardless of circumstances of birth. In the 1960's, the 'American Dream' was defined as a traditional family support system involving two legally married individuals providing care and stability for their biological offspring. Creating a 'Happy Home' was their primary objective. My parents produced two baby boys in quick succession. Available or acceptable birth control was not an option for the fledgling newlyweds anxious for the marvel of parenthood. Both at the ripe young of age of 22, my parents had barely enjoyed the innocence and curious experimentation permitted as teenagers before they were committed to parental responsibility to their offspring from birth to legal adulthood (18 years of age at the time).

My father had no college education, but an innate cognitive ability to master the alien language necessary to communicate with what was at the time the most state-of-the-art processing machines free from human error in the world, providing data for the United States Air Force, ensuring our post-industrial complex nation dominance on Earth, post-WWII. My father's experience in the US Air Force was attractive and valuable to the most prominent American based company of its time, International Business Machine, who recruited this elite young man, my father, to be part of the freshman wave of android-like employees of IBM, promising him and his family the security and benefits of this titanic corporation. My father was laboring as a human computer engineer at the gigantic IBM headquarters in Poughkeepsie, New York. The building was larger than the Pentagon. The Hudson Valley town of Poughkeepsie provided sprawling countryside ideal for suburban development, providing new frontiers to the company's employees recruited from around the world to homestead in what once was just another forgotten town in the historic state of New York. Every one of our neighbors whose children I played with, attended well financed public schools from kindergarten through high school graduation, and become skilled at elitist athletic activities like bowling, swimming, baseball, golf, tennis, and sunbathing at the tony IBM Country Club, exclusive to IBM employees and their families, were my peers. Every Fourth of July, we exclusively enjoyed an impressive firework display as the army of IBM families amassed on the immaculate greens of the Country Club's extensive world-class golf course. Every Christmas, IBM children were invited to the County Club Gymnasium transformed into the North Pole with a Christmas tree as tremendous as the celebrated Rockefeller Center icon, an affectionate Santa, and mountains of wrapped presents, sectioned by age and gender, overwhelming the vaulted dimensions of the gymnasium, for each of us commercially inspired Christmas enthusiasts to politely collect, already expecting Santa to deposit mountains of presents under the perfect farm cut trees we each had in our homes on December 25th. Christmas was a spoiled children's fantasy, that even the most well researched documentary on the fabricated holiday can't diminish.

I had to forfeit my 'Babes in Toyland' themed bedroom at age five when my still youthful, sweet, and glamorous mother conceived and delivered the baby girl she had always wanted to complete our ideal nuclear family. I came to find out that my birth was a surprising disappointment when born not the gender she had wished for, prior to the realization of Amniocentesis or Ultrasound. Determined that her second child would be a girl, she had already picked out the name 'Roberta', and had to muster an insincere maternal glow as she was discharged with her oversized second son (I was 2 weeks overdue), who she had to name quickly as she was sedated for 24 hours as I lay nameless in the newbie nursery still waiting for contact with my natural mother until she regained consciousness. Weighing 98 lbs. pre-pregnancy after delivering her first born, my older brother, my mother weighed 140 lbs. on the day of my birth, burdened with a two-week overdue growing human as she waited uninterrupted by the medical community for the precious labor pains that indicated it was time for her to be transported to the hospital, where my mother chose to be highly sedated. I was not brought to my mother's recovery bed by a welcoming maternity nurse, but for what reason I will never understand, my mother was wheeled to the public baby zoo window to view me amongst strangers who were pointing me out as the 'stud' (10lbs.8ozs.) who would soon be springing himself out of the nursery and walking out of the hospital on his own. An impressive boast to my self-esteem, but to my young mother, this was the first of many public humiliations I cast on her via folklore as her confidant. She even had a hand knitted pink baby sweater for her expected baby daughter that I was outfitted in by my mother when leaving the hospital. Again, her words, via folklore. I was left to process this story and its relevance in my development from child to adult. The 'Babes in Toyland' themed bedroom was evidence that they were willing to accommodate my inherent Disney fantasies, but that only lasted 5 years before I had to forfeit my personalized private bedroom to accommodate my new baby sister. My bedroom of origin was made over in a 'princess-ballet dancer' theme for the prized new female member of the family. I had to concede sharing my older, estranged brother's 'WWII fighter plane' themed bedroom. Plastic model airplanes he had glued together from model kits hung by fishing twine from the ceiling, and deadly Air Force planes bent on destruction made their evil presence in repetitive patterns on the wallpaper, attacking the enemy in the room, me. No more zip-a-dee-doo-dah Disney 'Babes in Toyland' mornings for me.

I recognized my older brother needed special attention when I was required to attend intimate parent/teacher conference when I was not yet in kindergarten, with my protective mother demanding my older brother, Michael, her first born child, not be held back from instrumental 1st grade as the teacher and respective school had recommended. My diminutive and attractive mother made her case, ensuring that I would always academically grow up two grades behind my older brother, reinforced by the fact that I was already quite independent from parental intervention in early childhood development and when I was of school age as I was a natural academic, capable of producing good if not excellent accomplishments and grades without much effort. I learned how to get the grades with the least amount of effort, and never wanted to ask or need help from my parents. I was the kid in the middle who didn't require what I surmised was the entitled special attention my siblings obtained, and I internally relished this feeling of autonomy. I lived in isolation from the family unit as I fantasized, I was not really a blood member of this otherwise perfectly functional household. I would sit in the family station wagon, daydreaming and channeling secret signals to the rest of the world from my passenger window that I was actually a famous royal celebrity held hostage by the plain kinsfolk populating the car, and I was not to be considered related to any of them. I alienated my siblings. I carried silent grudges that I sometimes acted out on that would lead to me being the recipient of more disciplinary actions than both of my siblings experienced combined in the entirety of their stay in our home of origin. Discipline in my home was never violent, but it was still emotionally painful to be forced to sit in the dining room facing the wall until my father returned from his job at IBM programming computers all day, so that my mother could relate her interpretation of my bad behavior; ranging from selfishly controlling the programs broadcast on our recreation room television over my baby sister's "Mr. Rogers' Neighborhood" obsession, to surprise attacking my older brother with my metal erector set creations for no other reason than boredom and probably a deep seated need for attention. I was a creative child and did not require any help deciding which activities were going to be classified as right or wrong by my estranged parents. I built forts in the secretive woods behind our house without asking my father's permission when pilfering his workshop for tools, for which I was always scolded. I made my forts for privacy, and they were always transforming.

My art teacher gave me my first taste of narcissistic validation when I impressed her with a drawing assignment in 3rd grade, declaring me a talent that could formulate into an artistic career. I had visions of me wearing a beret as I painted landscapes on an easel on the streets of Paris. I became addicted to that validation. At one point during my middle-aged success while living a luxurious life in New York City as a hard-fought proud gay man in sobriety, my mother confessed in confidence to me (in other words, "don't share this with your siblings") that I was always her favorite child. She qualified that statement with facts immemorable to me like that I did not cry uncontrollably, I slept and ate on schedule, and I never demanded the special attention or financial assistance it seems my siblings both required and cost my parents in childhood as well as early adulthood that I never knew about or considered consequential. I was the classic middle child. That's why I was honored to have been legally designated executor of my parents' estate, validation that I would have liked to receive the day I was born, and as I acted out as a rebellious adolescent anxious to be rid of all family obligations and emotional attachments with impertinence. But it made me the man I am, and struggle with emotionally today. I paid a very heavy price to prove my independence from family, society, anyone who gets too close to my inner child, and sometimes I don't even like to kind to myself. I can be my own worst enemy. But I have gratitude for everything and everyone that has been a part of my rocky, roller coaster ride of my life so far. And I know they will always be there in the future.

CHAPTER 2
Adolescent Revolution

I resisted experimenting with illegal drugs until I was emancipated from my claustrophobic suburban home of origin, where every adolescent move I made seemed to appear in my distrustful parents' crystal ball. I tried to maintain a degree of privacy in and out of their home, but whether delinquent or innocent, it felt like my experimental teenage years were always under surveillance. It wasn't like I was a serial killer; just a normal adolescent anxious to preserve the status quo of "a rebel without a cause" by participating in harmless juvenile delinquent behavior under the frightening weight of male peer pressure. I had no friend, sibling, parent, teacher, counselor, therapist or mentor of any kind to articulate how I felt; like I was always playing a role model male actor in a dramatization of life, not sure and certainly suppressing the homosexual desires that in the 1970's were presented as unacceptable immoral degenerates by the media. So, I kept my daily existence as a teenaged closet case as secretive as possible, avoiding conversations that would lead to parental interrogation that I intuitively knew would never resolve anything other than make me feel like more of a nuisance to my parents. My half of the double bedroom I shared with my older brother was searched in my absence for evidence I might have secreted. My older brother did not incite concern that he might engage in risky teenage behavior that might lead to legal consequences. I resented that my mousy elder brother was such a "mommy's boy." My parents instinctively knew what and how I spent my time when off the family property. They were protective of my hopefully consequence-free future, but more concerned that our ideal family unit was not the subject of any negative attention by our neighbors. It was important that my parents were viewed as role models of the perfect nuclear family by the rest of the homes strung along the curves, hills and valleys of our idyllically rural address.

Being accepted as a normal teenage male by my membership in a neighborhood bike gang was a disguise to suppress the fact that I had stolen courageous peeks at the sexually posed naked men in the newly published 'Playgirl' Magazine; a dangerous temptation if I were caught at the local pharmacy that stocked this adult publication next to 'Readers Digest'. The courage to procure the magazine that I was too young, and too timid, to purchase or shoplift, to privately study the men beautifully photographed naked aroused me sexually, affirming what up to now only my imagination had been suggesting to me. I was a homosexual. I wanted to lay naked with a beautiful man with a penis, and that the sexual exploitation of girls I engaged in at public school, even with some older college women who found me desirable, was a farce. I relished the sexist support I received for my sexual reputation by the male student body, some older and athletically superior to me, developing into a confusing veil of male validation from the reputation of my conquests on these naïve women as more than just macho comradery. It was these very macho men who I wanted to cast my charm over, to seduce them to lay naked with me. But for a young man in high school to be sexually active with women was not discouraged but applauded. I dated older girls with cars who got my sixteen-year-old candy-ass into bars with live cover bands to employ my dance genius, and further booster my sexual acumen to other older male bar mates and bouncers. I had more heterosexual sex during my sophomore, junior and senior high school years than my older brother did before he got married. I came home with my first amongst hundreds of family trophies my athletically superior parents and brother were awarded when I won Prom King. I was the golden figurine on the top of that trophy with a crown, cape and scepter. I was a young man who felt more validation for winning a Prom King trophy that towered over all the others awarded to my estranged family for their athletic excellence. But that narcissism felt like the gateway to homosexuality, which like my Prom King trophy, seemed forbidden, unappreciated by my blood family, and not the attractive fantasy I hoped it would be.

The family ranch house I left at age 18 to discover Time Square and homosexual satisfaction is still inhabited mortgage-free by my recently widowed mother and my socially bankrupt adult brother, Michael. He found unconditional acceptance from my parents, while my father was still alive, who were relishing the rewards of their retirement, when he returned to live in what was once the "fighter plane" themed double bedroom he and I once shared in 1964. Unconditional love and sympathy to their adult son after a very humiliating divorce, would never deny my now proud grandparents of my both of my breeder siblings, one of their own offspring respite at their home of origin, even though all three of us siblings were ordained to leave for college upon successful graduation from high school, never to return. Inhabiting the now designated "guest" room that my mother had redecorated in a "Laura Ashley" country chic motif, my older brother got comfortable and had no ambition or pressure to limit his stay. He is still there, 18 years as a "guest", more assured of his long-term residence since my father's death to provide companionship and free labor to my widowed mother who has always relied on a man around the house. She has never left the driver's seat of her car to manually pump gas.

As college educated young adults each living our lives independent of parental support, we three siblings were to respect our parents' retirement of entitlement (golf and bowling leagues, intimate vacations flying to exotic locales after years of family-friendly station wagon driven destinations). Professional contractors have been employed to perform extensive household upgrades and structural expansions to the home my parents would never leave after achieving the American Dream of owning a mortgage-free home, bought when starting a family when still very young and broke; now paid in full. My older brother is once again living in a fiefdom of the matriarch that still rules the family kingdom. My independent and socially active mother is in her 80's with the vitality of a 40-year-old. My surrogate "man of the house" brother pays his keep by mowing the lawn weekly, shoveling snow from a treacherous and long steep driveway, and pays my widowed mother a housing subsidy likened to rent as she washes his white briefs as she did for her husband of 60 years. Backward social mobility. My spiritually damaged older brother never grew back the falcon wings to fly far away from the house of easy comfort and childhood memories to build a new nest of his own.

I am proud and fond of the beatific 1960's ranch house I was safely raised in, conscious of the lush property that is rare by today's modern housing developments, with expansive extensions that enlarged the original restrictive floorplan, and modernized renovations to enhance the middle class comfort it steadfastly offered the original family of five to satisfy my mother and our diverse multi-generation modern family as we gather at our home of origin for regularly celebrated family holidays and events; central air, cable access for the 5 televisions spread about the house to accommodate various programming interests, a gas flame artificial log in the unique two-sided fireplace that my mother can remotely control to instantly produce the warm charm of a perfect yule tide log year-round maintenance free, and a complete makeover of the living room my mother has insisted on every performing every few years, which includes new wall to wall carpeting and custom drapes to complement the new furniture. I started a tradition of presenting my parents with small exotic seedlings of trees and rose bushes that populate the setting on anniversaries and birthdays, which have all taken to the property by growing, fleshing out the once barren landscape of the newly built house acquired in 1960. This 60-year-old home persists as the dynastic vortex that I feel obligated to revisit seasonally for holidays and family functions, that now include funerals as well as birthdays and bat mitzvas. I thought I left behind this haunting institution which I anxiously escaped with unresolved resentments when relocating my life and possessions to a college dorm at SUNY @ Stony Brook at 18 years of age.

My journey to my home of origin produces an initial burst of warm emotions as it pops into view at the crest of the winding country road it impressively resides on. It is a scenic thoroughfare, with twists, turns, hills and valleys, with every residence on this residential street, initially a dead end cul-de-sac christened 'King Drive', provided with undeveloped woods past their property line, ensuring a rural and private estate that distinguishes it from dense housing developments with limited privacy. My family house is a welcoming structure that upon knocking on the front door like a polite guest announcing my sincere homecoming, but all good intentions and expectations inevitably melt into a pool of anxiety as I begin to drown in uncomfortable unresolved emotions after twenty-four hours, as the upgraded rooms and hallways of the house of my good upbringing become claustrophobically stifling to my enlarged narcissistic presence on these short albeit all too regular visits. Wisdom, therapy, substance abuse, and pharmacology have allowed me to keep the focus on myself at these multi-generational stopovers to my home of origin. By bookending my visits with constructive escape plans like arriving in a rental car, reserving a room in a local hotel, establishing a healthy relationship with a man I present as my life partner who accompanies me giving my choice of lifestyle as much respect as my legally married siblings with kids. My long-term companion, Storm, is considered part of the family unit. I no longer feel like the fifth wheel at the crowded dining room table with nothing to offer in conversation, as the infertile gay uncle who doesn't exactly fit in. I arrange visits to acquaintances in the area to find validation and some respite from the crowded family home to during my stay and treat myself to a local luxurious hotel room to ensure my adult privacy and respite from the pressure to always be upbeat around the family. I do these things as if bookending a blind date, to preserve the otherwise proud dignity I owe to the security my home of origin provided me consistently from my childhood, and because I anxiously fear the rebellious adolescent emotions that become demonstratively immature behavior that begin to surface.

As sands from the hour glass empty after a full day with my family (regrettably I sometimes resort to alcohol in a bottle that is emptied by me alone, suffering the physical and emotional price of a relapse in an otherwise "dry" household), I regress to the rebellious adolescent monster who swore good riddance to my childhood home and the dumb-downed suburban town I had no pride, joy, or saw any future opportunities. Upon emancipation to college, I decorated my dorm room reflecting my unconventional personality with a wallpaper of empty Salem cigarette packs and another wall ironically devoted to the photoshopped beauty of the 'Playboy' Playmate of the month centerfold which I would study for its artistry, my middle finger waving like a ceremonial gesture upon my escape from the stifled bedroom of my youth.

My so-called angst riddled adolescence was in retrospect quite quaint. I ran with a gang of neighborhood boys on bikes, too anti-establishment to commit to extracurricular afterschool activities like organized sports or other special interest clubs. We male neighborhood compatriots united by boredom and bestowed with bicycles spent our days meeting up on the property of a local elementary school, IBMville, built specifically to accommodate the intense housing development of the same name, predominantly inhabited by the primary employer of this rural county, IBM. We took for granted that we lived in financially secure homes that could provide the homestead stability factor that some of our short-term school mates lacked, whose lives and futures were forever threatened with disruption because they were not lifetime members of the IBM establishment. Bicycles were our primary mode of transportation, and we all were blessed by our parents' generosity acquiring the Porsche of 1970's teenage bicycles, the 10-speed Schwinn facsimile of a racing bike produced in the post-psychedelic day glow colors of the era; lemon-yellow, lime-green, tangerine-orange. Garaged alongside our parents' contemporary and fully insured automobiles, we would unleash our trusty two-wheeled personal mode of transportation and independence as soon as we were free to leave the commitments of our suburban homes after school to congregate like a motorcycle club at the local elementary school playground before pedaling en masse from our all too familiar neighborhood to more populated areas of attraction, which before the advent of nationally recognized big box stores anchoring the social attraction of the indoor shopping mall meant grassroots mini-business strips consisting of banks, pharmacies, pizza shops, liquor stores, delicatessens, gasoline stations, craft shops, and barber and/or beauty salons. We may not have been financially savvy customers to these places of business, but we blended into the puzzle of local foot traffic that relied on their patronage.

Not tethered by occupational obligations or intimate romantic relationships, we were a gaggle of adolescent boys free and unsupervised to socially interact on a regular basis, bonded by our entitled ability to own and athletically operate a bike for hours a day to transport us to a variety of regular, and occasionally new destinations, as long as we were each at our respective homes' by dinnertime. We were all youthfully fit, and once we equipped our state-of-the-art Schwinn racing bikes with tachometers, the mileage and speedometer readings gave us a more quantifiable perspective on our nomadic lifestyle. Besides a few who had access to cigarettes, nobody seemed to need anything more stimulating or age inappropriate than to bike unsupervised with our asses attached to a 10-speed mass produced racing bike.

We biker boys, aged 13 - 17 years, were not classified as 'status quo' in our clique-oriented public school as none of us were proving ourselves to our family or classmates by joining any organized sports leagues. We were all very different, but the same when we biked in tandem. While there was the one customary magnetic cool dude, Sean, that we all secretly envied for his confidently immodest physical beauty, nobody in our posse was treated subserviently. We all got along, and we all thrived on good times. There seemed to be none of the social, competitive, or romantic drama witnessed at school. Once on our Schwinn bikes, we were like a grown-up motorcycle gang. Lawless, but loyal to watch each other's back. Positive peer pressure at period of sensitive adolescent self-esteem.

We trespassed around the suburban development of homes and surrounding undeveloped wooded areas feigning a delinquent attitude. A few six packs of beer were occasionally procured from an unsuspecting father's basement workshop. I never acquired a taste for the metallic can of bitter ale, which I surreptitiously poured the contents of into the earth behind me without notice. I never experienced the alcohol's buzz to establish it as a drug of choice. I did not want my peers to judge me as a wuss for wasting the beer and not getting wasted on the alcoholic content. It just was not my drink of choice.

Crafty associates of my mother's New England heritage handcrafted personalized Christmas stockings that we hung at bedtime on Christmas eve from childhood into adulthood, waking to find them overflowing with generous gifts that would keep us preoccupied as a family breakfast was prepared before the freshly-cut perfectly decorated Christmas tree in our living room was barely visible, surrounded by mountains of wrapped presents, courtesy of my young-at-heart parents and their thrifty contributions to a Christmas club account all year, justifying the lucrative spoilage. It would take hours for our family of five to unwrap the last present at the base of the tree, and a week to give each toy or apparel a trial run.

When I was 13, all three of us fortunate and spoiled siblings found a small alcoholic beverage, different for each of us, in our pre-breakfast and overwhelmingly generous Christmas stocking. My sister was 7 and had a bottle of Bailey's Irish Cream. I was 13 and received my first of what would become my drink of choice for life: Harvey's Bristol Cream. It is a syrupy sweet cordial that was promoted on TV by a sex-ready actor Billy D. Williams. I drank the then popular cordial that only English nuns seemed to possess, procured to reward their pious selves with thimble size glasses once a year. As an adolescent, it felt like an innocent introduction to adulthood condoned and supervised by my parents as imbibing in some Christmas cheer. I can't remember any parental scrutiny of my alcoholic tolerance. Never a black out, no vomiting, no hangover. Just part of the best Christmas mornings any other 13-year-old was openly indulging in. As an adult, I can drink a 1.5 liter of Cream Sherry in a day, a large bottle, and not vomit, not black out and know that if company is around, my generous offer to share my nectar will be rejected. When I discuss this fact with other alcoholics, they give me the strange look that Cream Sherry would be my drink of choice. It is an acquired taste. And I certainly acquired a taste for it as my alcohol of choice. I would wear the same proud expression I perfected in adolescents to mark my individuality, like when it was important to distract my secretly suppressed sexual desire to engage with penises and not vaginas when in high school. I thank my mother for assisting me with this important stage of adolescent self-esteem. But I found a decent replica of the iconic Harvey's, a cheaper and hard to find imitation, that I suspect I am the only customer who regularly purchases in my local customer friendly liquor store when I "relapse".

As a sexually confused and curious teenager, I snooped around my parents' bedroom for evidence of some sort of sordid activity. Most neighborhood homes I was a seclusive guest at had cocktail bars, 'Playboy' magazines, condoms, and once even an archaic silent black/white porn film that left me suspecting the parents of that household performed in. To my dismay and misrepresentation of my parents' sex life, they did not seem to require any stimulating devices. I scanned the paperback collection my en vogue mom indulged in, and even took the time to peruse the best-selling child rearing book broadcasting the unscientific childhood morality of Dr. Spock. I could not relate. I'm not too sure my mother put much importance in the advice from this common household paperback product. I was more engrossed in the best-selling "Doctor Reuben's: Everything You Want to Know about Sex but were Afraid to Ask."

As bad ass as my bike gang envisioned ourselves in our otherwise mundane adolescent lives, we never incurred any serious consequences until the summer of 1974 when I was 16. We took the illegal leap to acquire marijuana from someone's older brother. Most of us were in the frustrating age bracket of 15 to 17 years of age at the time, but we foolishly chose to experiment with this introduction to mind-altering substance cannabis on the bleachers of the local elementary school ball field, in plain sight of a meddlesome neighbor who called the police to break up our initiation to the illegal contraband before the party even got started. As the unexpected and unusual police patrol car approached the sanctity of our science fair project, experimenting with marijuana on the vacated elementary school property we roosted at, our gang disjointedly took flight on our respective bikes leaving the household plastic bag containing our virgin drug investiture in marijuana with the complimentary pipe resting on the bleachers as legal evidence for the responding police officer to package as evidence of unlawful and delinquent activity by a posse of criminals who had fled the scene of the crime. I circumvented my return route to the sanctity of my family home, surreptitiously blending into its insidious safety, nobody in my house the wiser that I was clearly rattled, when the very same invasive police car dispatched to the elementary school property was now a demonstrative presence parked on the curb of our innocent property to inform my pessimistic parents of my criminal and unmistakable pastime. The officer of the law facilitated an unprofessional intervention in our fashionably decorated living room. Our floor to ceiling convex picture window provided a fish tank view of the drama of our family's lives, where Christmas trees and new curtains broadcast our personal, albeit filtered perfect lives, so far not sullied by the presence of the innocuous law. The police officer and my estranged parents outnumbered me in my first intervention. I denied my guilt, pleaded innocent, and was left by the law with a soft slap on the wrist, but was forever branded by my misconstruing parents as the rebellious middle child who they foreshadowed as a lifetime drug addict that had already opened the foreboding gateway drug, projecting that I would soon be discovered in an innocuous closet with a hypodermic needle dangling from my venous arm with a lethal dose of heroin. My parents inflated this innocent rite of passage as proof that I was a degenerate on the path to a life of felony and criminal behavior. I never in my most adventurous episodes of drug experimentation was tempted by opiates. I never wanted to feel out of my narcissistic element by appearing intoxicated or overdosed. Opiates, specifically heroin, thankfully never became a temptation must less a drug of choice, and my parents now understand my chemical as well as my specific homosexual disposition.

After the relentless destruction of my 16-year-old human character, I was mandated by my hateful parents to an occupational commitment likened to judicially mandated community service; working at the predecessor of 'Burger King', a primitive fast food venue lost in business acquisitions known as 'Carroll's'. I was the 16-year-old resentful newbie who became submissive to grunt labor delegated to the least devoted member of the fast food manpower team. My older blood brother also worked at 'Carroll's' in a covenanted management position, delegating work but not contributing, enjoying his authority, and never showed his own blood brother, me, any mercy. I was disappointed that unlike what I saw in other families, my big brother failed me where I thought older brothers were meant to mentor you. Older brothers get in trouble, breaking the ice for when the next sibling repeats the same behavior, lessening the consequences. But we hated each other. I worked my lower class job obligations (working the shake machine on a busy Saturday was a fast-food disaster) to keep my overly disturbed parents content that I had structure in my after-school life until I provided physical evidence that my mandated fast-food sentence was producing unacceptable acne and back aches from the minimum wage chores even my brother did not have the backbone or the managerial seniority to spare me from. My mother could finally see the unacceptable consequences of my first, and last job in subservient labor. My material mother booked appointments with the best IBM approved dermatologist to perfect my skin as a reflection of her own genetic beauty, and allowed me to advocate for the pre and post college career I believed was worth punching the time clock for with pride: I became a Red Cross Certified Life Savings Instructor, advancing to Water Safety Instructor, to ensure top dollar salary and prominent social prestige employed as a certified guardian of the waterfront at summer camps with requisite room and board to escape living under my parents' "roof" during summer breaks from college, as well as the honor of mentorship to young adults who bestowed honest respect and esteem in my need for validity It was never a sexual thing, but I was sublimating my apparent lack of validation from my family, actually refusing to believe the discouraging projections of my bleak future (I was once told I would end up sentenced to prison, limiting my opportunities in life, and stigmatizing the reputation of our family) by designing a new approach to molding my employment skills, opportunities, and future without my parents' emotional or financial support. I also benefited from receiving the sexual appeal and approval from my peers and from my young minions, my swim students and summer campers who looked up to me like I was a god. I had a genetically perfect physique that swimming and boot camp calisthenics enhanced, and I felt like I was hired, played the part, acquired the validation, and mostly the narcissistic self-esteem to feel like the I was more than a role model. I was the superman I always dreamed to become. Forget about my tension filled home; I lived and worked at summer camps, with little or no family communication. I was emotionally independent of my family. And I was proud of myself.

I couldn't wait to escape the scrutiny of my unfulfilling adolescence, so I orchestrated my acceptance to Stony Brook University, known as the 'Berkeley of the East': a 'party' school. My parents wanted me to attend one of the many colleges further upstate that had top shelf reputations' as schools for engineering, but I was not interested in furthering my education in Math and Science; I wanted to explore my attraction to the hedonistic lifestyle that made an indelible impression on my pre-teen fantasies in 1969: 'Rowan and Martin's Laugh-in' and Woodstock. I was only 10 years old at the time of the popular mod comedy television program and the much publicized concert staged not far from my home, but I fantasized about being a free-loving, turned on/tuned out hippy with long hair, not afraid of drugs or nudity, much less working an uninspiring job just to make a living.

In the early fall of 1976, my parents drove me from the home that I had outgrown in Poughkeepsie to Long Island, depositing me and my footlocker at my Stony Brook dormitory. They drove off fast without a goodbye, good luck, or advice. We had not exactly gotten along during my adolescents, and they were honestly glad to get me out of their home, just as I was determined to exercise my 18 year old freedom in a progressive environment (no strict dorm rules—in fact, no supervision, no rules), and because I knew that I wanted to explore my suppressed homosexual desires in the city that handsome men from around the world were drawn to: New York City, only a two hour ride on the Long Island Railroad that conveniently stopped only half a mile from my Stony Brook dorm. Geographically, Stony Brook University fit my profile for 'college of choice' precisely to its proximity to New York City, putting the kibosh on any of the more prestigious colleges my parents dreamed that I would attend, locating me further upstate than the town of Poughkeepsie I had plotted to escape from.

My suitemates at Stony Brook, and most of the enormous University, procured marijuana in large bulk, for sale and to recreationally smoke, in our college suite living rooms until everyone was as lifeless as a zombie. I joined into the bong circle to interact with my peers, but decided marijuana just wasn't my choice of drug. I found myself restless rather than chill and didn't know what to do with myself in the stoned haze of the tranquilizing drug. Pot was officially on my list of drugs I could just say "No" to.

On my first day at Stony Brook, when I should have been settling into my new University life, it was more important for me to take the LIRR into New York City to troll around the area that I recognized as a sexual playground where my censored sexual interests would hopefully be satisfied: X-rated Times Square in 1976. It wasn't long before I was picked up by a humpy Italian young man, Tony, not much older than me, who detected my solitary presence as a naïve hick who needed a mentor. I experienced my first to man-on-man sexual encounter with a professional male hustler who took me to a seedy hourly-rare hotel for a gentle (no penetration) introduction to gay sex. I learned that Tony was also a stripper at the Gaiety Male Burlesque Theater, a secret gem for gentlemen who preferred the naked male physique in a more upscale establishment than most of the other tawdry all-male adult entertainment venues. The Gaiety, with a tasteful and discreet awning over the entrance bearing its name, was nestled between the respectable Lunt-Fontaine Broadway Theater and an authentic Howard Johnson's restaurant. Tony had an agenda besides tricking with an innocent young man like me wandering nervously alone in Times Square; he was scouting for a possible addition to the diverse line-up of men the Gaiety Male Burlesque

Theater offering their clientele diversity. The patrons of the Gaiety in 1976 appreciated more than just the chiseled, hairless, "gay for pay" male strippers, the "straight" male dancers, that would later make Chippendales successful. There was a variety of types stripping at the Gaiety when I debuted there: macho, fem, of all nationalities, who performed various choreographed and costumed performances that satisfied the range of sexual tastes of the audience, and truly represented the Gaiety Male Revue as Broadway Burlesque Theater. I was the young stud 'fresh from the farm', amongst the street savvy men who had grown up fast under difficult conditions in the big bad city. I came out on stage not in an uncontrived costume of the simple street clothes that an 18-year-old in 1976 would have felt comfortable in: flannel shirts, jeans, and construction boots. My hair was cut long in the fashionable feathered look of John Travolta. I was given the stage name 'Xristo' and introduced as the "All-American Boy Next Door."

I did not have any hesitation about stripping on the well-lit stage of the Gaiety Theater to an audience of demanding customers (strange men and an occasional woman), as I had always sought validation while growing up in the suburban town of Poughkeepsie. Not so much self-conscious but concerned with what my peers (primarily popular attractive classmates) thought of me, I concealed any indication of my true sexual identity while in high school by dating and having sex with many women, some as much as two years my senior. I knew how to dance unlike most men (read: heterosexual), so I made women happy on the dance floor which continued in the back seat of their cars. While in high school, I only wanted to feel like a handsome young man who was sexually active, keeping my homosexual desires a secret, and was doing what was impressive to my male peers by dating and deflowering many anxious female classmates. But it was the handsome young heterosexual male classmates whose validation of me as a virile stud was my true desire as their "locker room talk" meant more to me than all the young female hearts I broke. It meant the world to my suppressed homosexual desires that I had the admiration and respect of my male high school peers, but I was seriously suppressing any misinterpretation of my authentic intentions.

I saw college as more than just a chance to further my education and bolster my career opportunities for a respectable future. It was my ticket out of the small town and small minds of Poughkeepsie, New York. Without high school peer pressure and out from under my parents' 'roof', I conquered the forbidden act of homosexual sex, and with an experienced, young, muscular male hustler who dispelled my misconception of how undesirable homosexuals were presented in society. Tony was only one or two years older than me, and in his street tough, uneducated Italian way, I was not expecting gay sex to be something I would enjoy. But Tony was the perfect gentleman with my sensitive homosexual virginity (again, NO PENETRATION!). Living closeted at home upstate, I had to make do with the photo images of naked men posing in 'Playgirl' Magazine. As seedy the hotel room in Times Square was that my virgin gay encounter with Tony took place, I will always remember how natural it felt to lay naked in bed with a muscular macho man who was much more appealing than any of my male high school classmates. And Tony knew how to sexually satisfy me, and I was excited to reciprocate. After we both climaxed, our paid one hour in the hotel room was over, and I did not know where this romantic date would go from there.

Tony explained to me that he had to hurry to get to the Gaiety Male Burlesque Theater, where he was as a paid stripper, and induced me to come a-long. I had already gone down the rabbit hole of gambling with my sexual morality, so I dutifully followed him to the Gaiety, where we were buzzed in by the well-groomed middle-aged Greek divorcee owner and manager of the all-male establishment-the Gaiety Male Burlesque Theater in the respectable theater district of Times Square. It was my first VIP treatment. Tony led me down the dark aisle of the surprisingly opulent theater while a primitive gay porn movie was in progress. He sat me down in an aisle seat and told me to just watch the show. Suddenly, the movie came to an abrupt halt. Rolls Royce's hit song "Car Wash" replaced the overly exaggerated moaning of the male actors of the porn film in progress, the stage lights came on to reveal a performance arena with a long runway that extended through the center of the theater, and a silver Mylar curtain was drawn to cover the movie screen, making the stage look like something fantastic was about to happen. I could now look around the theater to study the audience; mostly older men (40 – 70 years of age) seated alone, a few groups of chatty giggly younger men happy to be in the company of friends, a few women nervously wondering why they were there, and one awkward male/female couple. The MC announced the '4:00 pm Gaiety Male Burlesque Review' was about to begin over a public announcement microphone from the movie projector/DJ booth, reciting the lineup of names which only mattered to some obvious regulars who were excited to clap and cheer when the name of a dancer they favored was mentioned. Otherwise the atmosphere in this particular Broadway theater was subdued bordering on shameful now that the audience was no longer under the anonymity of a darkened show palace.

The first dancer came on stage, did an unimpressive impersonation of an S&M Leatherman to Donna Summer's "Love to Love You, Baby", and left the stage to polite but discouraging applause. He obviously did not excite anyone, certainly not enough to be rewarded with any monetary tips customarily thrown on the stage.

Tony was introduced next as the "Italian Stallion" to enthusiastic applause and cheers from the regulars in the audience. Tony gave them just what they wanted. While porn star Andrea True chanted the disco hit "More, More, More" that exploded from the Gaiety theater speakers, Tony appeared on stage wearing nothing but his jeans which contained a noticeably restrained bulge in his crotch. Tony didn't dance to the music; he simply approached each and every member of the audience stationed by the stage, and teased them by stroking his engorged crotch, until he ended the torment by releasing his "Italian Stallion" cock to satisfy the audiences' expectations. He never took his jeans off, but only lowered them down to his hips, and left the entirety of his routine to his famous cock. Still not dancing, his only movement was to shake his oversized hard penis to the left and the right, slapping the engorged member against his hips like a metronome. This simple, and confident, routine was a crowd pleaser, as Tony was showered with monetary tips, some delivered personally to the stage by admirers not seated close to the stage, all of which Tony had to sweep up as his song and his act ended.

I was confused that the Tony, the man that I had just spent an hour intimately exploring each other's naked bodies, was now being shared with the general public in the Gaiety Theater in Times Square. But I was still a naïve hick, experiencing pangs of juvenile infatuation. Tony suddenly appeared by my side, crouching down to have an intimate conversation with me still in my designated aisle seat, while the third dancer in the revue was already performing on stage. Tony persuaded me that I could get up on the Gaiety stage, and become a professional stripper, just like him. This was a far cry from my winning 'Prom King' only four innocent months earlier, while still a sexually confused senior in high school. But Tony, who I had so far trusted as my mentor while aimlessly wandering around the dangerous temptations of Times Square in 1976, convinced me that I could do this. I was not only willing but eager to gage my validation with the Gaiety audience.

Music was quickly picked out (the Ritchie Family's hit "Best Disco in Town") in the DJ booth, Tony rushed me through the private door to the backstage dressing room, and I was coached on how to satisfy the audience as he caressed my adolescent penis until visibly hard in my jeans. Tony had convinced the DJ to cut me into the line-up of scheduled dancers, so before I had time to get nervous or check my hair in the dressing room mirror, I heard the DJ introduce me as a new dancer, 'Xristo', to the opening prelude of "the Best Disco in Town." It was like I had practiced for this moment all my life. It came perfectly natural for me to dance free style, expose my body which I had always been obsessed with developing and exposing, while performing a decent dance routine unrehearsed to the music, with tips and a roaring applause for my virgin performance as a stripper. And I was sober.

I had satisfied Denise, the owner and manager of the Gaiety that I would be a welcome member of the professional male dancer lineup. I stripped on the stages of the Gaiety on weekends from my classes at Stony Brook and supplemented my wages from stage dancing with personal performances in the many hotel rooms and private homes of gentlemen who wanted to pay for my intimate and expensive company. I was a professional stripper and male hustler from 1976 – 1978, lucky to not incur any consequences (legal, medical or physical) while I continued to attend Stony Brook University, graduating in 1981 with a Master of Arts degree in Public Affairs. I also learned to develop the muscles on my body, eat blueberries to increase the production of semen for multiple daily orgasms, and discovered how my mind could become sexually aroused in any environment when clouded with the toxic chemical aroma of "poppers"—amytal nitrate. I was a graduate of Stony Brook University with an education in exotic male entertainment and sexual escorting.

Most of the other dancers at the Gaiety did not have the healthy upbringing and future opportunities that I had in my favor. Yet, most of the street savvy strippers were eager to offer me a place to sleep, took me to the best underground clubs that I would not have the knowledge or the nerve to enter, as dance clubs kept a low profile, not advertising their business to the general public, employing intimidating bouncers that let only a particular caliber of patrons into these exclusive clubs, admitting what was considered acceptable patrons to keep the club elite: celebrities, drug dealers, drag queens and gay men. Many disappointed heterosexual couples were told that this was a "Members Only" club when rejected admission. Embellished by the company of other young and attractive Gaiety dancers who had been enjoying entre to underground clubs while still young teenagers to escape the ugly reality of their lives, the growing hedonism that disco music and clubs around the city were offering got me easy and complimentary entrance to a world far from the enormous indoor malls that were now the focal point of recreation back home in Poughkeepsie. I was now part of an elite population that discos sought to fill their large dance floors with confidently underdressed and physically fit gay men who knew how to dance enthusiastically to the long sets of mixed music that the DJs could keep drug fueled patrons dancing non-stop for hours. Very little conversation was necessary; it was all about feeling the music and expressing yourself through dance. Body & Soul.

My Gaiety street savvy co-workers also provided me with many drugs that I would maybe never have experienced if I didn't leave Stony Brook for NYC every weekend. Acid and Mescaline were an easy and cheap way to keep me stimulated and enthralled for the long nights dancing to the trippy disco music in the dark underground clubs that kept late hours. But I soon found my drug of choice: Black Beauties, which would give me the high-energy to dance and talk non-stop, so that sleep became a low priority while performing over my three day weekend commitment to perform at the Gaiety and continuing to dance recreationally until dawn at the best underground clubs in NYC. Disco music became my sole significance for the next 25 years, and the drugs that I relied on to keep me energized on the dance floor changed each season like fashion.

I lived a dual life; stripping, hustling and clubbing on weekends, but determined to graduate from Stony Brook on schedule. I was ready to trade the illicit lifestyle that NYC represented for a legitimate corporate career. With my resume highlighted with my acquisition of a graduate degree (read: no reference to work experience), my professional job opportunities expanded, and respective salaries escalated. With more disposable income, my progressive drug of choice evolved from the 'stimulant du jour': Cocaine, MDMA, Ecstasy, Crystal Meth. Alcohol was always a necessary chaser. By 2002, twenty-five years after my first nude performance at the Gaiety at the fresh age of 18, I found myself unemployable at age 42 due to my preference to party all night on alcohol and drugs than maintain a respectable professional job. Because I kept myself in great physical shape (narcissistic fear of losing my looks was more important than being gainfully employed), I was hired by a male stripper production company to be a go-go dancer in clubs throughout the tri-state area driving extensively in my unreliable but eye-catching vintage car, a rare orange 1973 Volvo 1800ES Sportwagon, that I pimped out for picture work. I still had what it took to satisfy the booker of the male stripping production company, and the clubs were satisfied with my performance. While the money I made covered the expense of keeping a high-maintenance mode of transportation running, and the alcohol I could not start the day without, the biggest perk was the availability of crystal meth provided by the production manager booking me who was always on-site to keep the his posse of dancers sexually motivated with the insidiously dangerous crystal meth to satisfy the fantasies of the paying audience. Crystal Meth became my drug of choice. It became my cause to live and to die.

CHAPTER 3

Recovery Culture

After successfully graduating with a Masters' Degree in an accelerated five-year program from Stony Brook University, playing house with my perfect peer and lover, Fernando, and dodging the dangerous consequences of the illicit lifestyle I had engaged in at a potentially instrumental moment in my life as a naive 18 year old Times Square stripper and escort, I developed into an independent adult devoted to promoting my new professional attributes; my graduate education, my lack of any record of criminal activity, and my well-honed presentation skills for securing a prosperous career in successful corporations in NYC. I studied the Thesaurus for 'word power' well after execution of my SAT exam. I took a summer job at the progressively sartorial downtown fashion establishment 'Barneys' to enrich my 'Macy's' non-designer level wardrobe. And I had been perfecting my humble charm and my formidable genetics to transforming my cute but flawed high school facade into movie star quality, like I saw my young parents.

I was fortunate to have encountered Fernando on the dancefloor of the Underground, the club of choice for local New Yorkers to frequent on Thursday nights before the chaos of Friday and Saturday "bridge and tunnel" mobs inundated the city streets and clubs. The Underground was on Broadway and Union Square, in one of the many buildings in what was still an ungentrified area anchored by Union Square Park that had hosted one of the many incarnations of Andy Warhol's factory. Fernando and I met physically on the Underground dancefloor, where I could discern whether a handsome stranger was worth pursuing for sexual intimacy based on dancefloor chemistry. I you can't dance effectively with me; I wouldn't put any faith in our sexual dynamics. Fernando passed, from the dancefloor, our first communication at the bar, in bed in my Brooklyn apartment (I wanted the upper hand in this immaculate encounter), to morning breakfast on the Brooklyn Promenade sharing our mutual and inclusive dreams and goals in 1981, at a time that gay men were still relishing their sexual promiscuity pre-AIDS. But Fernando and I were in agreement on our desire for a committed monogamous relationship. I was 21, finishing my last semester in grad school at Stony Brook, with a deadline to submit my Masters' thesis while Fernando had been working and paid very handsomely with perks as a flight attendant in what was still an exclusive and well-paid career as a tri-lingual male flight attendant for the premiere airlines in the world: Pan Am. The only other iconic international air carrier still maintaining the same level of service was TWA, with its architecturally important terminal at JFK, a bit more preposterous than the more befitting Pan Am terminal. Pan Am flight attendant uniforms were designed by Adolfo. Ralph Lauren for TWA. Competitors, but more powerful to survive the dwindling airline industry had they become accomplices.

Fernando and I kept our ambitions manageable, acquiring a promising and enormous parlor floor apartment in rough and tumble Fort Greene, the weakest in the hierarchy of the Downtown Brooklyn "brownstone triangle" that included the perfection of Brooklyn Heights and the opportunities and security of Park Slope. But our first new home was a palace, and we lived, decorated with antiques, and entertained many small and large scale parties in this diamond in the dust of a neighborhood defined by its proximity to deadly Bedford Stuyvesant, Downtown Brooklyn, and the crack epidemic with no incident to our home our persons for the 12 years we lived there. Fernando and I had the same dreams and goals, building a domesticated life in an incomparable homestead and bountiful lifestyle shopping and traveling, advancing my financially profitable career while never giving up my obsession to recreationally party: drugs, clubs, dancing every weekend.

At one point I was challenged by Fernando to see a therapist, a science for life we both respected, but I had yet to entertain until I was chastened for my increase in alcohol consumption. I did not feel threatened as I felt perfectly within the limits of my recreational substance abuse that was shared with my partner. I regarded the weekly visit to various therapists as a luxury item to compliment my prosperous lifestyle, like joining a gym I would commit to use regularly, visiting a Dermatologist for elective surgery (read: skin peels, Botox and laser treatment to eliminate sun damage and acne scars to perfect my most self-deprecating feature, my skin), or investing at an insider's price in an apartment as a building was going co-op in a yet to be gentrified neighborhood. At the time, the health insurance provided by my employers did not recognize therapy (or gyms memberships and Derma-tology) as important enough a medical practice to ensure productivity in the work place, so I would have to include the cost of the 40 minute sessions every week in my budget as I had to pay out of pocket. This fact tarnished the intimate dynamics between my therapist and me, as I resented the thera-pist pontificating on the importance of regular appointments, which meant regular payment by me, even if the weekly session was cancelled by me in advance due to a personal, business, or recreational conflict. The therapist seemed to be prioritizing their guarantee of my business income before their concern for my general welfare. This unappealing domination combined with the belittling I felt I received from these seemingly discontent profess-sional social workers (I never could afford a licensed PHD) would eventually lead to my executive decision to terminate the business arrangement, citing dissatisfaction with my feelings and ethics of my blessed life always being scrutinized and minimalized. The persistent focus on my timely devotion and energy I devoted to body building, what I always believed as a healthy fitness activity that also built my self-esteem, was interpreted as wasteful narcissism, as per their intellect. As they put it, bodybuilding was not neces-sary to maintain a strong muscular body unless it was utilized in an occupa-tion demanding heavy manual labor. None of my therapist seemed to at-tempt to identify with my inner soul, and I was paying for their services! I guess I assumed that as long as I showed up on time for all our regularly scheduled appointments with payment in hand, I should receive some valida-tion from this paid mental health professional. Almost a reversal of my experience as a paid escort. But of the handful of therapists I engaged with from 1981 – 1991, not one of them seemed to make me feel better about myself, and damned if I did not try to charm them. In retrospect, I can say that from my first consultation, when I frankly and boastfully shared the details of my lifestyle, the red flag of my substance abuse was raised, but I was unaware or inclined to disparage any part of that debatable issue in my life.

In all my adult years recreationally partying on an array of mind-altering substances on a weekly basis, I was still advancing in my high-demand line of work professionally and financially. I never felt I had a problem. "Weekend Warrior" was the title used to not stigmatize a hard-working, hard-partying professional. As long as I wasn't arrested or charged with a crime while on my party time, my job and career would remain intact. I could not allow the two incompatible lifestyles that feed off each other to overlap from playtime into office time. I had to maintain a bookend to the dual personality of the two clashing worlds I lived in. I had to and would be back in the office Monday morning clean and sober to perform my job duties until the end of the work week with no complaints from my employers. TGIF.

I was never diagnosed by any of these mental health professionals that I employed with a mental disorder, apart from narcissism and alcoholism. As much as I honestly shared and justified my usage of mind-altering substances as if it was just part of my gay culture and club lifestyle, I would be deeply offended by the therapists' stigmatizing diagnosis. That was not why I sought private therapy, and I was not ready to give up my predilection to use drugs and alcohol to enhance my hedonistic lifestyle. And the persistent conflict on bodybuilding that the therapists' view was unnecessary in my office vocation, not requiring manual labor, and their general attitude that its significance was purely narcissistic.

I was never offered a prescription to any psychotropic medication during the ten years I played therapy patient whore with various MSWs. I usually gave the therapist a two week notice that I was going to discontinue our sessions (a good professional ethic), so that the last two sessions would be a trial by the therapist of my escaping the core "truth" that the therapist, like a mystic, sensed was coming to the surface of their crystal ball and I was a coward to face it. I interpreted this frantic confrontation as the therapist's last-ditch effort to guilt me into reversing my decision that would leave a void in the therapist's datebook and regular income.

I magically prospered in the corporate world, acquiring new jobs with advanced titles and enormous (25 – 50%) advances in my yearly salary without making any effort beyond taking the blind faith of an employment headhunter who would know of my credentials to cold call me like a gypsy reading tarot cards, already forecasting my willingness to produce a current resume to accompany me to an already scheduled appointment to interview for my certain next new job and fast track career.

Burson-Marsteller was my third job since college graduation, making 125% more than my first job ten years earlier upon college graduation, in 1981. Burson-Marsteller was the most successful and largest Public Relations firm in the world, making millions creating the buzz words "Just Say No" to enhance the image of the reigning First Lady, Nancy Reagan. My salary was obscene considering what little I was required to do and the lack of pressure or responsibility on the job. Lunch hours turned into alcoholic revelries with willing derelict coworkers confident that there would never be any trouble once we returned to the laissez-faire attitude of our bosses and the company as a whole. Returning to the office alcoholically buzzed, I would page my cocaine dealer for the powder substance that would wash my vodka cloud away, reignite my alcoholic pilot light that would pull me back out to cocktail hour like a strong undertow, and get lost in the deep dark sea of decadent New York City clubs open seven days a week, and finally drown in the party binge when I would pass out at 6am to wake at 8am for another day of work and substance abuse. It was hard to keep wading above the flotsam in the drowning pool of my life, but the hubris of my arrogant mind made me continue day after day, week after week, year after year. My liquid lunch coworkers stocked beer and liquor in their mini-fridges, desk drawers, and credenzas. I found familiar folded glossy paper manufactured to secure cocaine origami style on the rarely used stairwell in this recently renovated multistory landmark building in the newly revitalized Flatiron district. It was 1991. Burson-Marsteller was at the top of their game. My tunnel vision and deaf ears prevented me from the oncoming economic storm that would intervene in my career's life, and many otherwise undeserving members of the booming economy.

I had learned that the best night to party if one lived and worked in the city that never slept was Thursday, making Friday at work a difficult feat to muster if you drank, did drugs, and did not like to leave a club until the DJ started losing his populace. On one particular Thursday night, my 2nd boyfriend (more like a boy-toy as I was recently "divorced" from Fernando after a record 12 year relationship, in a midlife crisis at age 32, and Gustavo was only 21, of Cuban descent, a souvenir I acquired on a drug fueled trip to Miami, pre-South Beach, who followed me to NYC to experience the incomparable nightlife with the man who knew how and where to party) and I took Ecstasy to better enjoy a campy chic disco party hosted by a European faux underground socialite, Susanne Bartsch, who held parties at various off-the beaten-path locations. On this particular night, the Susanne Bartsch party was held in the historic but sadly ignored Copacabana nightclub. As we descended the stairs to the subterranean dance floor, disco pop star Alicia Bridges was standing on the landing, spiky bleached hair, halter top, silver lame skin-tight jeans, and fuck-me heels, singing in a loop her one and only hit song:

"I like the Nightlife; I love to Boogie."

I like the Nightlife

I love to Boogie

Under the Disco Ball . . .

I don't know how long she had to sing that same silly song that night, but it was like something you'd expect from a party for people who would appreciate the camp of hiring a one-hit wonder to perform like she was at Studio 54 fifteen years earlier when the song was a commercial hit. Now she was stationed alone on stairwell, lip synching in a loop, like some automaton in Disneyland.

Gustavo and I returned to my newly acquired East Village Co-op some time before dawn. As my boy-toy dropped to the bed capable of sleeping like a baby, I wrestled with the speed portion of my Ecstasy gestation, making calculations as to how many hours I could squeeze out of the alarm clock before having to get ready for work. As the sun rose through my eastern blinds, I realized I needed to cut the edge that the chemicals and my own internal anxiety were fostering by slipping quietly out of the apartment to buy a six-pack of tall cans of Budweiser; 6 tall boys to keep me company during the end of my Thursday night party as my boyfriend was no company as he did not suffer the same post-party-insomnia as me. By 8:00am, I knew I was not in any condition to go to the office, and called to tell a young staff member already on duty that I would be taking a "sick day", which I had already taken a lot of that calendar year.

At 9:30am my work pager went off, indicating that I had to call the office. I was told by same young staff member, who I supervised, that I was to report to the office. The messenger's voice was nervous, as if he did not relish giving me, his boss, this message. I reminded him that I needed to take the "sick day" as I was truly "sick". The messenger's voice dropped to a whisper as he pleaded that he was only following the orders of my boss, who demanded that I be in the office by 10:00am. I did not have a good relationship with my boss. I don't think he respected my professional performance, and I avoided contact with him even on a "normal (sober)" day. It is a fifteen minute walk from my co-op home to the office, giving me no more time to groom without a shower, brush my teeth profusely, take a last final racehorse piss to empty 5 of the six tall boys I had consumed, wake and alert Gustavo that it was time for him to go to his job, and blubber that I feared I might not get out of this binge gainfully employed.

An eerie stony silence met me when I passed the normally gregarious security guards in the lobby of the PR firm, which continued as I walked down the hall to my office, passing my boss's closed door, nodded at one of my drinking partners from the previous day's lunch, and checked in with my own small staff on duty, both of which looked at me with the same nervous fear that I detected in the messenger's phone call only one-half hour ago. I retired to my office.

I was the System's Manager of the computer room with a loyal staff of 9 computer operators working 3 shifts at the notable PR firm. My office was decorated with more pieces of funky art than most colleague in my profession would deem appropriate. Retreating to my office to await my execution, I tried to log onto the computer system that I was responsible for managing, and found my desktop computer was not responding, as I was locked out. Foolishly, I reproached the female staff manager who I had assigned the responsibility of account maintenance. She looked like she was going to cry when she had to tell me, the man who had hired her for this job, that she was following orders from my boss, and that she was truly sorry. I still was not sure what she had to be sorry about, as the sense of entitlement I had that gave me the tenacity to get drunk during a work day, and have cocaine delivered to the office, did not allow me to believe I was getting fired from my coveted job for what my defensive mind was minimalizing as a rare circumstance.

The fact that my "sick day" was already disrupted when I was instructed to appear at the office, albeit an hour after the 9:00am start of business day, and locked out of my computer by my own staff, preventing me from performing my usual morning duties, given no indication by my otherwise loyal staff and co-workers as to what was going on, made me indignant enough to march, still quick inebriated, down the hall to knock on my otherwise difficult to approach boss's door. I was hired four years earlier by my current boss's predecessor who must have seen some potential in me to perform the managerial job that I held for the last two years that paid me good money. That man who promoted me, who I respected and had a good business relationship with, had since left the firm, to be replaced by a bald headed, villainous mustached, ill-dressed man who I never got along with, who was now instructing me to return to my office where I should do no work, but just sit and wait for his call. 10 years of career advancement and now I was in the principal's office facing serious consequences.

What little alcohol was in my system to otherwise medicate me had now evaporated from the increasingly anxious adrenaline coursing through my chemically imbalanced central nervous system as I returned to my silent office cell knowing that I was about to be fired, probably for the obvious truth that I had a drinking problem that interfered with my ability to function at the capacity my judgmental step-boss deemed acceptable. I wondered about how Alicia Bridges felt when she was paid for her gig last night to portray herself in her glory days for a party of people probably too young to even know or appreciate who or what she was at Studio 54 in 1980. I once had the professionalism to acquire this and other prestigious jobs in New York City when I arrived fresh from graduate school in 1981. This was going to be the first time I was going to lose a job, and the fact that I just HAD to see Alicia Bridges perform while on Ecstasy the night before rather than get a good night sleep to arrive at work sober and on time seemed foolish in retrospect. I lost my indignation as I worried about how my career and my financial future in New York was going to be destroyed, humbling me from the otherwise charmed sense of entitlement that fueled my career and reputation. There was also my newly acquired mortgage and maintenance on my 1st real estate investment, my co-op in the East Village. My job seemed like a low-priority next to my desire to drink, drug, love the nightlife, and boogie.

I was finally called into the ugly step-boss's office and asked to close the door. With a very stern and disapproving look, he instructed me to sit. I was sure this meant I was getting fired, and possibly a slight intervention if not a lecture on how he saw my substance use effecting my professionalism. The meeting was started by a third party in the boss's office: A Human Resources executive who did offer the solace I was so looking for. I was told that due to the poor economic forecast looming for the entire national business world, our company was down-sizing, and I was selected as part of the first wave of lay-offs. I still could not accept the thought that I was now no longer wanted by the firm, and directed a query to my boss first, and then the Human Resource executive as to whether this was due to my attendance, conceding to the fact that I had tried to weasel my way out of coming to the office this very day. While my boss sat silent, I was assured that this was an economic decision by the professionally objective Human Resource executive whose job duties included facilitating awkward firings and layoffs. I knew I was overpaid for what little services I rendered. There was no need to put up a defense.

I was offered six months of full salary severance pay intended to allow me to take some time and evaluate my life, my career, my relationship, and my substance abuse. None of these topics were explicitly mentioned in my lay-off, but it was implicit to me. After the Human Resource executive presented me with my severance package documentation organized in a folder, I was escorted from the building as per protocol, and I walked home from Union Square to my lower East Side first-time property owner co-op that I had only occupied and paid one month mortgage on, stopping at a local liquor store to buy a bottle of bargain friendly Svedka Vodka, the generic of the name brand 'Absolut'. This reminded me of a morning when I was rushing to my job in Union Square, and I saw a well-dressed thirty-something young business women pushing her way through the two old glass doors that served as the entrance and exit for this same established liquor store that still had a neon sign electrifying the word "Liquor" in a urine yellow hue. The alcoholic cosmopolitan girl I spied on emerged from the lower Park Avenue Liquor store, grabbing the neck of a bottle bearing an unfashionable brown paper bag to disguise it. I took in the image of her as if I would need to report the details to some authority after it was reported that something tragic happened to her, with pleas for assistance in case of her disappearance, as if I was the last to see her alive; high heels, attaché case, shoulder purse, trench coat, wisps of blonde hair flying lose around her face, Union Square, customer at Union Square Liquor Store. If I had to describe to the concerned authorities what expression was on her face, I'd say it was a combination of anger, shock, worry, and a little satisfaction that she was able to obtain the medicine her emotions hungered for at 9:00am. I assumed she had already been to the office, received some upsetting and unsettling news regarding her employment prognosis, and was now predictably heading home very early with a bottle of booze to keep her company for her first day unemployed.

Now it was my turn to play the entitled loser.

I was home again with my own bottle of alcoholic unemployment, Svedka Vodka, and my severance package folder. My boyfriend Gustavo was still in my home preparing for his normal day at work. I guess being 21 years old makes the "morning after" not so devasting as when you are 32 years old and had suffered through regularly scheduled unabated hangovers for 14 years. The relationship with my boy-toy was already rocky, and one of the last vestiges of my dignity to his young impression of his "daddy" (he was a 'shop boy' in clothing retail), was my well-paid professional job that I now no longer possessed. Instead of tackling my new unemployment with a rolodex of loyal network contacts, I came home with a bottle of vodka, and an immediate phone call to my cocaine supplier to tackle my drug addiction by feeding it, which did not impress him.

Family, friends, lovers, employers, and the clubs that I frequented never called me out on my behavior. I was a functional substance abuser. It was important for me to maintain an appearance of absolute control while in clubs and bars. If I felt that my alcohol consumption was making me feel sloppy, I'd straighten up with a stimulant. If too much of a stimulant made me uncomfortably anxious, it was time for more alcohol. It was a roller coaster ride. I felt like a mad scientist trying to balance the disparate effects two disparate substances. If insanity has been defined to me as repeating the same behavior to suffer the same unwelcome results, I wanted to know why it seemed like only I could not be happy with just being a falling down drunk, or, a tea-totaling coke head. Why both afflictions? If I avoided both substances, I could be in that neutral point of mind that I paid so heavily to chemically and alcoholically attempt to achieve. It was a roller coaster ride that I could never seem to be satisfied with.

Then I was introduced to Ecstasy. That replaced Cocaine as my drug of choice. Like in the corporate world, the real estate market, boyfriends, parties, and clubs, I was always granted privileged drug connections. The pharmaceutical pill's active ingredient, MDMA, produced a false sense of euphoria, where everyone in the vicinity of the user of the drug was embraced with chemically induced love. Ecstasy was actually manufactured legitimately by pharmaceutical plants and prescribed by licensed marriage counselors to eradicate the wasteful conflicts of patient couples during sessions to produce a more respectful and empathetic settlement. But just like any legally prescribed pharmaceutical medicine discovered by the drug-hobby population, the USDA realized the dangers outweigh the overall benefits, stopped production, and any surplus stock is was sold on the black market. I loved the first few months of indulging in Ecstasy, gladly disposing of all the negative elements of a night of cocaine consumption. But just like every other drug of choice, I would become a glutton, and take many more pills than anyone else I knew, and certainly more than originally prescribed by the medical community. I suffered debilitating Sundays, bedridden the whole day, moaning and groaning to my then boyfriend after partying on a diet of Ecstasy and Margaritas from Thursday through Saturday night (breakfast, lunch, dinner, and long nights out in the clubs) like the desperate and dramatic opera character Camille, who personified for stage the suffering from consumption, like my consumption of Ecstasy.

I was a bedridden zombie on Sundays, wrestling with how I had once again wasted a weekend not enjoying the respite from my job and all the recreational activities that might have made going back to work a more restored employee on Monday, like most "normal" professionals engaged in on weekends. I would lay paralyzed by anxiety from the excessive amount of poison, lack of proper nutrition, and sleep deprivation after three consecutive nights of partying. The anxiety mounted as Sunday night evolved into early Monday morning. I dreaded the doom that I had to be at my job by 9:00am Monday morning to assume the sober responsible professional appearance and performance I needed to receive the big paychecks that paid for my expensive lifestyle and weekends of excessive self-indulgence. AA or rehab did not cross my mind. I was in my early thirties and was struggling but not ready to admit much less commit to a life without hedonistic pleasures. I took care of my appearances, so from the outside I looked great. I was even scouted and mentored into a short lived and eye-opening experience building a modeling portfolio.

I strangely never thought asking nor did any of my therapists ever suggest that pharmaceutical medicine might alleviate my suffering: anti-depressants and anti-anxiety medication was freely dispensed in late 1980's, and MSWs could write the script. The subject just never came up in my sessions. I never disclosed the truth of my illicit drug use, or any feelings that would denigrate my exterior shell of narcissism to my mental health professionals. Besides the recreational illicit drugs, I consumed regularly every weekend for years, I also ingested excessive amounts of Tylenol PM to induce the sleep I so wanted.

My degrading and overly drawn out breakup with my boy-toy Gustavo ended gracefully with his eminent return to Miami, more as an exile from NYC who he had unforgivably burnt his bridge with. I was the best opportunity for both of us hot/hardheaded Taurus/Leo narcissists to start afresh.

On my own volition, I enrolled in a local outpatient substance abuse program as my severance package was reaching its limit, allowing me to still maintain my freedom to live in my home and successfully land a new job in New York City while attending and successfully completing the 5 month substance abuse program that motivated me to remain clean and sober for five years. I surprised my family and friends that I was still able to partake in all the same nocturnal activities that I loved and relied on free of abnormal substance enhancement. I would set my alarm clock on Saturday nights to arrive at the after-hours clubs at the insane but peak hour of 4am to dance until noon on Sunday. Because I loved to dance in good clubs for long hours, even sober, I could still reach the nirvana I had thought could only be achieved by juggling various mind-altering substances all night, and usually through the next day. It felt empowering to no longer be a slave to substances, and still achieve the euphoria that dancing through Saturday night gave me.

I always had a coterie of other friends in recovery who did not want to miss out on the fun of clubbing, and I felt relieved of the aching distraction to find the next right boyfriend. Surrounded by friends was more fun, and I found porn to be an efficient substitute for romance. Late one night at the Sound Factory, the dance club of choice after the Paradise Garage closed, I won the attention of an exotic, masculine man of the world who was impressed with my sobriety, established career, and lack of any scandal in what gay social circles he inquired about me. I had what was called "good credit rating". After four sober years I did not trust my instincts that meeting the next man in my life at a club producing the fantasy world of escapism gay disco provided as a dangerous prospect. Our initial awkward conversation in the surreal "never land" of the nightclub 'Sound Factory' impressed me that he was a man of high standards, so when this intelligent Persian (read "Iranian") proudly held my hand in the streets of New York after a few regular and escalating dates, I was smitten and naïve to overlook the predictable conflicts would that would erupt when two strong minded Taurus's would battle over dominance. What I was really naïve to the fact that my Middle-Eastern lover, newly transplanted from San Francisco, was a regular user of Crystal Meth, as it was the new drug of choice for gays, who relied on the substance to be transported from the west coast to feed the barren meth market now growing in New York City, which I fortunately got clean and sober before crystal invaded the gay drug culture. The insidiousness of this man-made drug in a mentally unhealthy mind (read homophobic) was a secret my new lover kept from me, and I was blind to the evidence that something was not right when my possessive and generous lover of one year would incite public and private arguments with me that would lead to his dramatic exit from a public restaurant or the comfort of my home, absent from my planned activities, and ignore my phone calls for days. Until caring friends starting wising me up to accounts of my lover's dark side, explaining his erratic moods and behavior and appearances in unsavory venues I could not fathom did I realize I was being manipulated by this man I loved into behaving like a pathetic masochist, not a role I ever saw myself performing. I refused to believe the stories of my lover's sordid sexual behavior acted out in public when we weren't going through the motions of our mutually agreed upon committed relationship: holidays, visits to my family home, vacations, even a mock wedding at a counter in Tiffany's to secure his citizenship. Once I had heard enough of what I first thought was jealous gossip, I confronted him, and learned the truth. I felt like I was in a three-way relationship which I still believed I could conquer, but as friends and family took pity or a leave of absence on this unending saga, I would not give up on "fixing him" as I could not imagine life without him. I loved him. I read up on everything I could learn about Crystal Meth like it was a science project I wanted to successfully win, and switched my regular AA meetings that I attended for my peace of mind and began to attend Al-Anon meetings shifting the focus from my own recovery to how to save him and his destructive substance abuse for the sake of my pathetic fear of losing him and our so called relationship. Al-Anon meetings were not as structured as 12-step AA, and I found myself commiserating in the company of young desirable women as confused and hurt as I was that the one and only man in their life was a self-centered junkie who absorbed time, energy, and money from the one loving caring human being who could just not call it quits. We all cried, as we all felt this was unfair to such desirable partners as we saw ourselves, but pathetically could not save ourselves much less the addict we loved. Debby Harry was considered the icon of co-dependence by forgoing her musical career to care for her heroin addicted boyfriend for years before he finally succumbed to his disease.

After 5.5 years clean and sober, I never felt so mentally unhealthy in my life as those tumultuous years breaking up and making up with a meth head, I couldn't break free of. My friends and family got tired of the repetition of my recanting the latest drama story and began to alienate themselves from my soap opera life. One rare peaceful Sunday morning after a quiet weekend together, he broke the serenity by admitting he was suffering from acute withdrawal from meth, begged me to understand and allow him to score and return with the substance. I offered up my sobriety as a sacrificial lamb to keep him from deserting me, wanting to believe that maybe as a last-ditch effort to salvage our relationship both of us should be on the same chemical frequency. He hesitantly served me my first bump of crystal meth. Now I experienced what he didn't want me to realize: the insidious drug made me feel invincible, and my sexual prowess multiplied. The drug seemed to distort the reflection I saw of myself in the mirror; as if a fairy godfather had granted me a wish of perfect beauty in a distorted magic mirror; satisfaction with an image that only an hour ago focused on flaws. I was relishing our bond, but to sabotage this chemically induced experience relishing a new drug of choice in the comfort of my home, my inconsiderate and now nervous lover made plans to leave me alone so he could escape me, his guilt, and the repercussions of his decision to introduce me to crystal, and so he deserted me to find solace with his meth head friends, who I despised as much as they resented me. I had now discovered my newest drug of choice, 'Tina', who would cock block any further romance with Sharif, the flesh and blood love of my drug addled life.

My destructive lover left me to deal with this unfamiliar and scary high on my own. I never forgave him for that humiliating rejection. I never felt so manipulated by someone I was hopelessly in love with taking on the pathetic role of a masochist. I immediately obtained a bottle of vodka and ordered an eight ball of cocaine to reignite a relationship with my old and trusted friends in a bottle and bag who I had forgone for 5.5 years. Fuck crystal meth and fuck who I thought was the love of my life. My once respectable upscale lifestyle took a swift turn down-market.

I resigned from my six figure consulting job, sold the impressive co-op apartment I had just completed extensive renovations representing myself as an inexperienced but ambitious sub-contractor to cut costs and corners, so that the apartment sale set a new high for sales in the otherwise stagnant East Village high-rise. The proceeds from the cash sale allowed me to move into a quant but tastefully renovated Victorian home in my sister's hometown of Buffalo. The house was architecturally impressive, immaculately landscaped and situated on an enviable plot of land bordering a beautiful park providing the residence a peaceful respite view of a plot of nature from every household, with a discreetly engineered entry and exist guaranteeing privacy and a sense of entitlement. I had the cash to secure the sale with substantial down payment, left with more money to decorate the 5 bedrooms, living room, dining room and garage with a new Audi paid in full of cash. A "sweetheart" deal in real estate lingo. Arlington Park Inn. Indulgence in daytime television watching 'Jerry Springer' became a guilty pleasure with too much free time on my hands. Alcoholism blamed on boredom. Married to my gay sister, both of us on the rebound. We shared a sophisticated modern twist to decorate the 5 bedroom Victorian home even my parents were impressed with, but we had noisy disagreements over the most trivial of cohabitation: temperature control, the acceptable amount of time before a dirty utensil should be washed, the amount of time a vacuum should be allowed to interrupt the household, specifically during the broadcast of 'Jerry Springer'. We began bickering, then arguing, only to make up, like a married couple.

We opened our impeccably decorated home as a Bed and Breakfast, respectively called "The Arlington Park Inn". I never desired or found myself staying in a B&B, as I was drawn to the privacy and dark minimalism of boutique hotels. Now I was the owner of a business that violated my sense of privacy as strangers roamed my home beyond the boundaries of their bedroom, living and dining area. I did not think this venture through. I ended up relapsing from NYC and Sharif, leaving the B&B and home I had invested my life savings to furnish in the hands of my business partner and blood sister, relinquishing all claims to any financial profit from the proceeds of the property, art, and furnishings in my absence. Absence in person as well as in spirit. I was an addict to Sharif and his manipulative supply of crystal meth, as well as the resulting masochistic role is assumed and suffered emotionally from.

CHAPTER 4
Non-Elective Institutionalization

My out of control lifestyle crashed and burned on a frigid night in January 2004, a 46-year-old unemployable drug addict and alcoholic working for currency in the only occupation that did not require sobriety on the job, as a go-go man. I was desperately driving the last of my assets, a rare 1973 orange Volvo 1800ES Sportwagon to get to a last minute dance gig for pay, tips, and crystal meth, at the legal speed limit, but too fast on the dark winding country roads coated in treacherous black ice. I was in a drug trance, anxious get to a dance gig 3 hours away in a strip club in Springfield, Massachusetts. Without any warning, I lost control of my car on a curve and sat powerless as the picture perfect sportscar independently drove straight off a curve and down a steep ravine, tearing through weak young trees until the vehicle stopped at the bottom of a 100-foot ravine. I surprisingly walked away from the wreckage fortuitously with my handsome face unmarked, considering the consequences had I hit a solid tree projecting me out of the antiquated seat belt, smashing through the windshield upon violent impact. The police arrived on the scene of the accident, observed no external damage to my person necessitating any need to call for professional medical attention. I was not even asked if I had been drinking. I was at least 12 hours sober.

I walked away from what should have been the end of a tragic story; a 46 year old man dancing in clubs to sustain a daily drug and alcohol addiction,

as well as being technically homeless, totaling the last of my prized possessions; a rare 1973 orange Volvo 1800ES Sportwagon, the same car rewarded
to that year's Playboy Playmate of the Year, Marilyn Cole, in a special edition
painted pink. While I was welcome to stay in the home of my origin by my
parents who had forgiven and forgotten our family differences, and because
I had outstayed my welcome at all my rent responsible friend's homes in
NYC, and I did not want to overstay my welcome with my now retired
parents given my illicit lifestyle. I could always find many homestead options;
my cockiness always counted on there being a Plan B. I was generously given
access to many weekend retreats that my more ambitious hardworking
friends who continued to advance in their careers and their respective invest-
ments in upstate New York rural weekend real estate. Well past their middle-
age crisis, unlike me, these faithful and responsible friends no longer appreciated the value of partying and savored the stories I would tell about my
juvenile and happy-go-lucky life. At the time of my accident, I was living easy
by staying rent-free at the weekend retreat of a gentleman who liked my mess
of a presence around whenever he would return from a week of work in
New York City. Larry wasn't much older than me in years, but the fact that
all I did was lay around his house until I needed money/drugs/alcohol,
would I become motivated to drive away from him and his remote cottage
deep in the secluded hills of mysterious Pawling, New York to where ever I
was booked to dance in the tri-state area with no regrets for the way I used
him and his hospitality.

With no legal charges placed on me by the responding authorities attributing "black ice" as the culprit to the accident, I was a carless free man. I
bashfully told the police officer that I did not have anyone that I could call
to drive me home (I was only 5 miles from the cottage I was calling "home").
I got a ride back in the squad car to the dark and very remote residence that
the gracious Police Officer could not believe was an actual address, as the
private dirt roads in this undeveloped countryside were not registering on
the police cruiser's navigation device. Once the considerate but clueless Police Officer saw me enter the uninhabited cottage and switch on a few lights
to assure him I was safely home, he carefully backed up the rocky roadway,
leaving me without his knowing that I was far from safe and sound.

I was left alone at the only place I could call home to concede to the abandoned, reckless, drug addicted hole I had dug myself into. I no longer possessed the transportation necessary to get me to dance gigs to make money, crystal meth, and alcohol. The cottage was secluded and miles from civilization. I felt I had reached rock bottom, and there was no one that I could call to rescue me. The only way out of my predicament seemed simple: suicide, the first time I contemplated this self-centered act during what was once a fulfilling life.

After overdosing on what I thought were a vial of pills I found in my host's medicine cabinet, medication that I thought would anesthetize me into a peaceful lethal sleep, I came to discover my naive lack of knowledge and innocent unfamiliarity with prescriptive medication that devastating night. I had never been prescribed or taken any psychotropic medication in my life, so I had mistakenly swallowed a bottle of Wellbutrin, which is actually an antidepressant, based on the familiar yellow smiley face warning of drowsiness, and I woke up from my suicide funeral slumber in a psychotic rage that was further fueled by my aggravation that my overdose was unsuccessful. Unable and unwilling to get out of bed lead me to attempt to suffocate myself as my limbs seemed paralyzed by the Wellbutrin overdose. I tried my hardest to press my face into the mattress until I could see the bright white light of death, but always came up for air as I learned the hard way that self-suffocation is too easy to bail out of. I did succeed in bruising my nose, and leaving deep face prints on the mattress, further evidence for the Police Detectives responding to the scene of the crime to take note of in their investigation of my auto-asphyxiation that lead to more self-inflicted assaults to my person during this torrid nightmare, when professionals were dispatched to the lonely address to inspect and report on this homicidal crime against myself.

My third amateur suicidal act was to an attempt to hang myself using the railing enclosing the loft that the death bed was situated on. I set up a denim jean jacket as a noose, a chair to reach the noose below the loft, only to find this ridiculous, even in my desperate state of mind. I could barely hobble down the loft staircase much less climb up on the hangman's chair as my legs were not functioning from the paralysis from the Wellbutrin overdose.

Frustration was replacing my desperation to end the agony of my so-called life.

I was now left with the desperate option I had always remembered as the dramatically portrayed suicide of choice in movies. I sat in a filled bathtub armed with the large butcher knife I sharpened regularly for domestic duties in the kitchen, like slicing barbequed steaks, and began carving my wrists.

I lay in a lukewarm bloody bathtub, taking more determined hacks with the knife into both wrists like I was sawing two-by-fours of wood, until I felt the tendons and nerves sever like marionette puppets cut from their operating strings. The water had drained from the tub, leaving me bloodied, cold, and mortified by the hallucinations from the Wellbutrin overdose, horrified that I was no longer alone in the remote cottage deep in the woods, but that the property was being surrounded by townspeople with torches approaching the scene of my self-induced crime, peering into the cabin windows to witness my self-crucifixion. I suspect this was based on my recall of the influential classic movie "Frankenstein", the misunderstood and fatal life of a monster. I was petrified, naked, motionless and silent in the bloody cold ceramic tub, fearful of the power and the anger emanating from the imaginary ruthless mob gathering outside the cabin. This went on for hours, interrupted by bouts of vomiting and convulsions from the overdose. I could not understand why I was not yet dead.

The only movement I made while I lie paralyzed in that bloody bathroom were convulsions of dry vomit from the overdose, and the wonder of my enduring livelihood as I studied the self-inflicted severed wrists that were now like puppets without operator strings (the major tendons and nerves on both were completely severed), yet blood was not pouring out at the deadly rate I expected. I had not done my research on successful suicide, and as deep as the lateral wounds were, I missed severing the blood arteries that a Boy Scout with a college education and a Prom King trophy had missed out on ever researching the proper method of killing myself.

As the sun rose, I was shocked and annoyed by the unexpected appearance of two very genuine city visitors who unbeknownst to me had been invited to spend the weekend at the cottage, generously and unknowingly toting bags of overpriced culinary provisions from Balducci's to compensate for the chance to escape the brutality of living and working in New York City, only to discover a crime scene that they were more frightened by than anything that they would ever encounter in NYC. The two visitors politely announced their presence from the unlocked sliding glass doors that served as the main entrance to the cottage, coyly explored the uninhabited rooms until they came upon the gruesome site of me, naked, bloodied from head to toe, curled in a fetal position on the bathroom floor, hoping to complete my frustrating suicide hours after the executive decision to overdose after my car accident, now disappointed that there was to be an irritating intervention to what I believed to be the climax of my so-called glamorous life. The sun had risen on a new day in my so-called messy life.

At first appearance, what the two naïve visitors (estranged to me; I not only did not know them, but had no forewarning of their invitation to the otherwise empty house), and that they had discovered a gruesome crime scene presumed to be perpetrated by some brutal criminals on my innocent person. When they asked the horrified question of what had happened to me, I believe they were not prepared for the snarky tone in my voice declaring that I was trying to kill myself, and their company was not exactly welcome. I was frustrated and tired from the long dark night. I agonized over not pulling off a successful suicide, and now I had to contend with the unexpected saviors who were going to thwart what was proving to be an amateur and aborted crime against myself. I was the innocent human vessel possessed by a demon.

As I sat on the bed, comforted by a blood soaked comforter with the sun rising to announce a beautiful new day, I sat alone, as I had made it very clear that my saviors/unexpected guests were to stay away from me, which they obeyed my mandate as they seemed to be cooperating on the extended phone call to 911 until EMS arrived. It was then that I had a vivid, curious and yet obvious, even my altered state, was an apparition. I considered myself an agnostic (actually an atheist but found 'agnostic' in AA as less antagonistic with its vagueness to a Higher Power and invitation to explore your own form of spirituality), but I did not have a biblical revelation. As I sat defeated alone on the bed with the sun ending the darkness of the long night, I saw three Native American persons standing against the wall in the small bedroom adjacent to the bloody bathroom only 6 feet from me. A 30-ish male guitar player intensely focused on his performance on his instrument, a young girl, 8 - 10 years of age, with two long braids dividing her raven black hair and a simple dress smiling at me as children innocent of "badness" in the world often do. Lastly, I observed an elder Native American with long silver hair and beard, gesturing the sign of the holy cross, only backward, as I was familiar with the Catholic ritual performed by my father when visiting family gravesites. I was told by therapists and case workers that I should never forget the details of this apparition, and even did some research into the culture and rituals of my apparent visitors, who I was not frightened by, but actually shook my head to erase like an etch-a-sketch. I lost interest in discovering any secret message from this moment, but took it as a personal, unique sign that there is some spiritual force that visited and perhaps inhabits me, that has always been with me, perhaps thwarting the futile attempt on my life that night, and assuring me, inspiring me that I had more to contribute in life. Without subscribing to some bogus TV commercial projecting unconceivable ancestry from DNA, I had firsthand knowledge that my paternal grandfather's brother had married a Native American woman. I had more of an affinity for her culture's spirituality than my mother's Presbyterian Protestant or my father's Roman Catholicism.

Police officers, detectives, and EMS vehicles found their way to the reclusive address where the petrified and helpless weekend visitors stayed on the phone with the 911 operator, keeping their distance from my bloodied, naked and angry body. I felt I was possessed by a demonic manifestation and sat shivering and hallucinating spiritual images in the guest bedroom, keeping the human guests and the hallucinations at bay from offering me any comfort that I truly did not want. I believe I made it clear that they were interfering with my grand finale, and they got the message loud and clear that I did not welcome their presence much less their only option to be of any assistance to this debacle but to take authority over my obviously self-involved and failed fiasco.

After a preliminary examination was performed by the responding EMS team, and a frank interrogation of the forensic evidence after a methodical investigation of the rustic cabin by professional police detectives revealed that I was the culprit of various crimes against myself. I was strapped into a gurney (which given the dangerously icy conditions of the path from the cabin to the parked EMS vehicle was truly unnecessary given my ability to walk), and was involuntarily transported not to the nearby hospital in Sharon, Connecticut, but a long one hour ride back to the hometown I had left 28 years ago where my parents still lived, Saint Francis Hospital in Pough-keepsie, New York, which offered the orthopedic surgeons experienced with possibly repairing the severe damage I had inflicted on my wrists, which would determine the future functionality of my damaged hands. While I did not bleed to death (my blood had coagulated by the Wellbutrin overdose), I had severed the major tendons and nerves in both wrists. As I looked out the back window of the ambulance en route to the hospital, I could see the familiar roads that were taking me back to the town of my origin, which I thought I had escaped from when I was a frustrated 18 year old waving my middle finger as a gesture of "goodbye and good riddance". Ironic fate.

Both EMS attendees rode in the front cabin, leaving me strapped in a gurney for the hour long ride, as if I was going to bolt out the back of the van still bloody naked, not something I considered, but lonesome for com-pany on my virgin ride in an ambulance after my monumental failure at end-ing my life, which was a personal defeat what with my arrogance from inde-pendently accomplishing more than my parents expected of me in my independent life. I had succeeded in breaking a 6-figure yearly salary, owned and successfully profited from investing in three real estate properties, traveled around the world; all of which I believe irked my parents out of jealousy in surpassing their humble middle-class existence.

I didn't expect small talk while immobilized in the back of the van, alone, unattended, unheard. I would like to have asked some serious and specific questions regarding my livelihood. And couldn't I have been consulted as to which hospital I would like to recover at? Why, oh why?? Fucking Pough-keepsie!!!

This was not what I ever envisioned as part of my illustrious life. A Mas-ters' Degree in 5 years. A progression of job advancements not based on my technical skills but my charm, professional appearance, writing skills, and ability to patronize amongst a dysfunctional staff to keep corporate depart-mental harmony peaking at age 38 when I broke the six figure salary to retire from a career I never was interested in and a financially prosperous real estate sale that allowed me to make a life style change from the monotony of living in NYC for nothing other than the quality of discos. I had made the life change pre-40 that most Americans never get the opportunity much less the courage to do well past mandated retirement and benefits at age 65. I was the envy of my own parents. And now I was just a possession of the medical team transporting me to a hospital without even consulting me as to what and where I wanted to go, much less give me the courtesy of allowing me, a once prosperous citizen of society, to ask about my condition and my prospects for livelihood. I was a ward of the state. I no longer had any rights or privileges I had worked so hard to endow myself with. I had failed to end my life, and now I felt I no longer was responsible for decisions regarding my livelihood. I was a prisoner of a crime against myself. I was a failure sentenced to a life devoid of my ambitious independent spirit. I was spiritually dead.

CHAPTER 5

Highly Medicated Individual

I spent a surreal amount of time sitting upright on a gurney in the midst of the turmoil of the Saint Francis Hospital Emergency Room at dawn of a Sunday morning, in the very city I grew up in, always anxious to escape; Poughkeepsie, New York. Compared to sustaining a daily existence of crystal meth and alcohol consumption, this was fascinating live theater; the finale either life or death for the other souls who had suffered a traumatic Saturday night. I did not want to miss a moment of the hours I spent in the Emergency Room (3 – 4, but I had lost all track of time, day, and self). After a long sleepless dreadful night inflicting homicidal harm to myself, I never lost consciousness, but experienced frightening hallucinations that raised my adrenaline to quietly remain in a state of apathy, oblivious to the passing hours of darkness, in spiritual obscurity, naked and bloody on the cold tiles of the bathroom floor or curled into fetal position in the drained blood-stained bathtub, or enfolding my naked bloody cold body with a comforter pulled from the bed in a guest room in the remote suicide cabin that provided isolation from the sober world, deep in rural Pawling, New York. The bottle of Wellbutrin I misguidedly consumed kept me in a state of suspended animation, and the preliminary first-aid addressed by the ER team was to treat me for the overdose by commanding me to drink three very expensive bottles of liquid of "activated" charcoal ($700./dose), containing an intensely high level of carbon-rich materials such as wood burnt at a very high temperature to create a porous substance with millions of holes and crevices to increase the ability to bind with toxins in the gastrointestinal area, thereby absorbing the overdose of drugs. No more stomach pumps!

But while the activated charcoal drink was caking my internal organs from possible damage from the excess of pills I later found out was not a sedative capable of producing a deadly sleep, but a popularly prescribed mild anti-depressant, as toxic as a strong cup of Starbuck's coffee, it also was also inducing violent medicinal vomiting. At $700. per bottle times three, my drug addict alcoholic mind was disgusted with the materially expensive waste. My severely severed wrists were superficially stitched up like darning a pair of over-worn socks to be dealt with later by a neurosurgeon who would assess the serious internal damage impairing the use of my hands and fingers. I felt like some kind of biblical character cloaked in nothing but the bloody wrap I had absconded as my only material possession from the cabin, which did not seem to be a concern to the orderliness of the Emergency Room. So, I drank my toxic tonic, vomited into a bucket, and waiting an hour for my next meal of activated charcoal. An overdose requires patience, with nothing or no one to interact with. Sleep was not on my agenda. I wanted to experience as much of this surreal moment in my life, sitting upright on a gurney in an ER, a first for me, like any first memory to store in our brains for future reference. While an impersonal nurse regularly checked my vitals, I was alone and aware that I was now no longer on Death's door experiencing hallucinations of angry townspeople or ceremonial Native American Indians. I was surrounded by trained life-saving professionals, supplies, and equipment providing triage to first level of care at a hospital. I felt useless, stationed on my gurney, just taking up space and time in the Emergency Room, Saint Francis Hospital, City of Poughkeepsie, State of New York, United States of America, planet Earth, the vast galaxy beyond, ad infinitum. It was like the singular incident of a bad acid trip I had experienced when I was 18 years old, naive to the dangers of ingesting chemicals, swearing to a foxhole god that I would never take acid again in exchange for some salvation from the frightening loss of reality I was not prepared or willing to go through on my own without praying to an entity that contradicted my atheism. I prayed for valium. I later learned that being an agnostic would grant me that genie wish.

As a fan of mind-altering substances, that bad acid trip taught me to appreciate the banality of feeling normal, and when I am content but restless, I try to remember that experience; feeling just plain normal should not to be taken for granted, but quietly and soberly enjoy it. That's what I channeled during my indefinite stay on the gurney in the Emergency Room.

The only article of attire that I wore as I was eradicated from the crime scene was a bloody bed comforter. That is all I had to comfort my naked, blood caked, temperature-impervious body hours later in a modern hospital in Western civilization. A variation of Stephen King's "Carrie"; once a gorgeously styled celebrated Prom King, now a detached bloody mess that would scare a popcorn eating audience. It was my shroud, my scarlet letter, my potential burial garment that no one from the crime scene attempted to remove from my alienated person, as if it was holy and not to be confiscated from pathetically lonely crazy self. I was treated more like a corpse removed by EMS with as little disturbance to the forensics at the crime scene even though they had the homicidal maniac in custody. Like an insecure infant, I desired physical as well as emotional comfort my bloody blanket was the sole provider of. I must have projected a very protective "leave me the fuck alone" karma to anyone who witnessed me on that bloody Sunday.

While I was a patient in the Emergency Room being treated for what the hospital deemed life threatening ailments, I was interviewed by administrative staff for information that any hospital would classify as standard procedure, but I found an invasion of my privacy. I was obstinate. I would not provide any contact information, specifically "next of kin". I did make it clear that I possessed no iota of medical insurance, which I'm sure was a more pressing matter to the hospital administration than reuniting me with my next of kin. Like all other circumstances that I encountered in my adult life, good and bad, starting with the day I was emancipated from my home of origin four months after my 18th birthday when I was driven in suppressed silence by my timeworn parents to my assigned dormitory at Stony Brook University, I never asked or was offered any emotional or financial support from my parents. I was determined to be the master of my universe. Although my soberly produced, proofread, printed and signed suicide document was addressed to "Whom It May Concern", my parents were assigned by default the recipients of my few surviving assets: my unconditionally comforting senior citizen Persian cat who was always by my side, and my prized vintage car preserved since 1973 with no imperfections until my unexpected life changing detour from the road I was expertly operating it on while innocently driving to my drug and dance destination. I would not provide the ER staff with my parents' names, address, or phone number, as I did not want my estranged elderly mother and father to be burdened with the responsibility of my hospitalization, emotionally much less financially.

Once I was released from the war zone atmosphere of the Emergency Room, I was placed in a private room in the Intensive Care Unit, the room barely big enough to contain the single twin-size sanitized infirmary bed practical for medical purposes but uncomfortable for the patient as the only furniture to rest on 24 hours a day for the next 7 days. The room was strategically adjoining the nurses' station to keep a vigilant surveillance through a picture window like the interrogation room in a police station. My suicide categorized me as a "high risk" individual, no longer a free citizen to make decisions for myself. Suicide is considered a crime against oneself, making me a ward of the state. The mini room had its own toilet like in a jail cell, offering no more privacy than a curtain hung with commercial strength rings to be easily manipulated open or closed with the jerk of a no-nonsense nurse's hand. Lastly, there was the constantly distressing alerts emanating from a cluster of technological processors that took up the majority of the ICU room, each with a respective monitor screen scrutinizing my vital signs by means of a multitude of wires attached to various parts of my body. An android life support system machine was my master as I was reduced to be a human puppet on strings. I had lost the liberty to live free or die. I was at the mercy of the hospital, contained in my private life support ICU room. It was no longer a free spirit predisposed to experience the endless wonders of life on Earth. It took a few days in ICU to adapt to the institutional rules of the hospital, realizing that I would never to be given a moment of privacy that my entitled and so far, consequence-free life had allowed my rebellious and independent spirit. I was assigned a gang of around the clock non-licensed medical employees, all of which were newly migrated to the United States from one of the multitude of Caribbean Islands that offered easy to acquire entry-level medical certificates providing them with the opportunity to work and prosper in our "Land of Opportunity" with very rudimentary nursing skills (operating a bed pan) and never even mastering the English language to provide constructive communication with their assigned patient. These women were paid to babysit me, performing no other tasks relevant to the hospital then to ensure my livelihood (prevent an expected subsequent suicide attempt), oversee my toilet use sans le privacy curtain, and offer insincere small talk, which I learned to ignore. My biggest problem was their lack of professionalism. I would wake up from numerous naps in my ICU bed wired to persistently alarming personal vital statistics machines to find my infirmary bodyguard engrossed in a daytime soap opera on the television at my bedside. The tiny television robotically positioned from a ceiling crane was not a complimentary perk in the ICU hospital room, much less the entire hospital. It was the property and jurisdiction of a for-profit enterprise not affiliated with the hospital and required daily payments to receive broadcast reception that my father generously paid for in advance for my entertainment. To wake up from a nap to find the hospice worker employed by the hospital engrossed in the tiny TV set positioned for her personal attention echoing the hollow script of a daytime soap opera incited me to behave like an arrogant, entitled lord scolding her salaried maid for insolence. I told the woman who I had no allegiance to her or the job that the hospital had assigned her to perform, that the TV was not for her entertainment, and that she had disturbed my sleep. After that incidence, I was categorized as "high maintenance". But I was beginning to tire of my institutionalization and was starting to recover my self-will.

When I first arrived at the Emergency Room of the hospital devoid of any possessions, specifically the contents of my man-bag (wallet with ID, cell phone, male hygiene like lip balm, blemish neutralizer, hair balm, cigarettes, and preparatory drug paraphernalia). I do not know if and who may have recovered my wallet containing my Driver's license as ID, but I resolutely remained "mum" when I was interviewed for the details of my empty life. I never revealed the names of my family or friends to the hospital staff as I did not want to involve my parents in my personal mess. I thought I would remain a "John Doe" to the hospital, and hopefully leave with no one knowing about my ordeal. But my driver's license broke my anonymity.

It was at this juncture of my 24-hour odyssey when I was dumbfounded by the appearance of my parents, conjoined like Siamese twins, at the doorstep to my medically ornamented room in ICU, politely and considerately waiting for me to acknowledge their presence. They were not going to cross the threshold to my limited domain unless invited. Very respectful, given I was trapped, and had nowhere else to go. I was unprepared and did not know what to say other than graciously appreciate their concern and their attendance, as bewildered and unexpected as it was to lift my veil of secrecy. My parents, after their immediate horror at being informed what is considered one of the most disturbing communications pertaining to the livelihood of their offspring, probably rehearsed how they were to best confront their middle-aged middle child institutionalized after a gruesome night of self-inflicted mutilation. I presume the were also prepped by a hospital counselor on how to best approach this unprepared for moment in their life as parents to a child who had given up on his. To my surprise, my once challenging parents did not confront me with the expected interrogation of my motive to bring this nightmare to a reality in our otherwise perfect family. No "Why??? Oh, why did you do this?". There simply is no straightforward answer other than a rhetorical "I'm Sorry!?!". Instead, I was awestruck, unable to construct a statement to verbalize during this awkward moment. My father, always short but succinct with his conversation skills, summed the moment up perfectly by acknowledging my feelings of frustration by declaring "You must have been very angry with yourself", alluding to the violence that I had sustained, and to have failed to reach my goal. He was right. I was always very frank about my low threshold for violence and bloodshed, fictional and real, so even I could not believe I resorted to the mutilation that I inflicted for hours on my wrists, and the disappointing failure that left me bedridden in the Saint Francis Hospital Intensive Care Unit for my parents to hopelessly witness. My Prom King trophy was no longer my Saint. My cold callous heart was melting with humbleness. I was damaged goods.

But I was not prepared to hear my mother describe her "lovely" visit to my secret hideaway turned crime scene in Pawling, New York to recover my cat and personal belongings (clothes, toiletries, and a laptop) as "a lovely property", hosted by the sympathetically courteous and helpful landowner and my enabler, Larry, not to mention that she qualified my sex-for-rent landlord as "handsome". That seemed inappropriate, awkward, and debatable. I resented the polite merits of Larry as a distraction from co-opting the reality of my current state of affairs. But following the pleasant script my parents had been coached for this epic conversation with their post-suicide son, the goal was to maintain a gentle atmosphere of forgiveness. My parents were novices at handling the nuances of polite conversation, dancing around the facts of the severe crime perpetrated by their son, a member of a stoic New England heritage, as far as we knew was pristine of any history of violence or criminal behavior, much less a son who they could never seem to be on the same frequency as, from infancy to middle-aged hospital patient. Perhaps the prepping provided by the hospital guest counselor on appropriate life-affirming conversation awkwardly qualified as socially safe banter, but my mother's remark on how handsome Larry was nothing more than a statement of opinion I was never planning on addressing in my lifetime, as Larry was not only NOT the object of my desire, I found him to be an angry, bitter human being to be a hostage in the company of, much less reside in his house and his bed. My father, sober 30 years but classified by the 12 step cult as a "dry drunk', was always a man of few words but never censored, flipped the reality switch on this socially, emotionally and perhaps legally sensitive moment were now standing with a sufficient space cushion before their emotionally and physically damaged son, being about as benignly considerate as vase of flowers delivered in thought but not in presence. It had only been a few hours since my parents received the insidious phone call from the detectives who between my cell phone and driver's license were able to track down my parents and relay through the medium of telecommunications the facts of my otherwise private affair.

My father looked deadpan, emotionless and with no body gestures to embellish his simple statement to me, his middle son, strapped to a gurney with a dozen alarm-producing machines encircling my bed, all attached to me, fresh casts immobilizing both arms from bicep to knuckles, my crowning Scottish glory of a full head of ginger hair freshly and unflatteringly shorn off and dyed black in a bored tweaking mistake after staring at myself in the mirror to long, synonymous with crystal meth binges. Under normal social situations, my mother would have demeaned the change to my appearance. But under these unusual circumstances, all that mattered was that we three were alive and present for this moment. I wouldn't have wanted this unannounced visit with my now no longer estranged parents to have played any other way. There was no guilt or apologies or uncontrollable words, emotions, or tears to clean up after they finished the formality of checking in on my resuscitated life. It was the first impression I sincerely felt from my parents that regardless of anything, they loved me. Having said what they may had prepared and rehearsed in the short car ride to fulfill the surreal obligation of visiting a hospitalized child, they left me in minutes to allow me to recover, while a background of busy in constant motion filled the dramatic scene with realistic extras like in a movie. But after my parents left, I reinforced my will to not become a dependence on my parents, as I am responsible for who I am, how I got here, and what I do with the rest of my life. Then I had a good cathartic burst of tearful sobbing, convulsing in the ICU unit about the reality of all of the events leading up this moment where I can't reckon with the pain I must be responsible for inflicting on my parents, two fine humans resourceful enough to know that this is not the end of the world. The breaking news of that day couldn't be any worse in their wildest dreams, but they would unconditionally provide the emotional support to help me get better. It's never too late to make amends with family.

After surviving my suicide, the hospital's resident Psychologist visited me at my ICU bedside. I bestowed an instant respect for this woman simply because I had never been professionally treated by anyone with the advanced academic title of PhD, and because I was desperately lonely and anxious for some intelligent conversation while chained to the ICU hospital bed alone, with the exception of my subservient Caribbean bodyguard. I was ready and humble enough to honestly reveal the lifestyle I had lived and loved for over three decades to someone who I considered intellectual enough to understand. But within that first meeting, the Psychologist diagnosed me as 'Major Depressive'. She really never listened to me. She was just following the protocol she was trained and hired to perform in this hospital to anybody that has done what I did to get there. I've come to learn this is a standard diagnosis for anyone hospitalized under my circumstances; a perpetrator of a suicide. I was prescribed and willingly swallowed a multitude of psychotropic pills every day, all day, morning to night, to hopefully neutralize the mental disorders that so far, I had self-medicated with recreational drugs and alcohol; anti-depressants, non-narcotic anti-anxiety pills, and sleeping medication. In addition, Neurontin was prescribed to alleviate the throbbing pain in my hands resulting from the self-inflicted severed tendons and nerves from sawing my wrists. The pain in my hands was further complicated by the tender neurosurgery performed to attempt to reconnect the severed tendons and nerves. My hands are like twin crack babies that throb and ache when overused at the end of the day, which I can blame on nobody but myself.

My question as to why I was transported by the responding EMS team from the reclusive scene of the crime in Pawling to a hospital in the home town that I thought I was liberated from 28 years ago, Poughkeepsie, New York, instead of the closest hospital for life saving emergency treatment in nearby Sharon, Connecticut, was beyond my understanding and my jurisdiction. It turns out that the thorough EMS team responding to my condition made the professionally thoughtful decision that Saint Francis Hospital in Poughkeepsie had a very reputable Orthopedic Surgical team, specifically the renown genius of the most difficult neurosurgery cases, Dr. Bravados, where the damage I had inflicted to my wrists could be addressed, requiring microscopically meticulous surgery to reattach the major tendons I had successfully severed, and possibly recover some of the multitude of nerves that were also in need of attention. Serendipity. I was meant to return to the home of my origin.

My first visit with Dr. Bravados was days after I had languished in ICU. The esteemed surgeon visited my bedside to assess the damage and was not an opportunity for me to charm the esteemed Doctor like I had learned to do all my life. I spoke only when instructed, and his lack of bedside manner must have been an indication of his self-arrogance. His brisk entrance to my private room in ICU was shadowed by the respectful acknowledgement of his fellow hospital colleagues who may never have met the Doctor but knew of his reputation. His stoic immodesty of their acknowledgement of his presence did not soften his bedside manner. He was a narcissistic prick, not interested in any pleasantries. I could have been Robert Redford (younger), but to him I was a cadaver in need of his services, which he was accredited with being top in his field in the North East United States. He gave a preliminary examination of my damaged wrists, gave no consideration to my personal well-being, or the patronizing hospital staff star struck by his presence, and barked to whoever was responsible that I was to be scheduled for neurosurgery in 3 days. His parting words to me were "I can't promise any long-term reversal of the damage you have inflicted to your wrists, affecting the future use of your hands", or something along those discouraging lines. As far as the severed nerves, he gave me the textbook explanation that nerves were inoperable; like earthworms that are severed, they continue to function, and may actually reattach, but that was out of his hands and up to chance. And he was right. My hands, specifically my fingers, are as compromised today as before Dr. Bravados' acclaimed six-hour neurosurgery. I have only 40% utilization of my fingers and hands. The severed nerves limit my dexterity and ache like I have a permanent case of frostbite. I have learned how to position my hands in public so to not bring attention to the stigmatizing scars.

The three days before said surgery were filled with blood work to determine any allergic reaction to the anesthesia, MRI X-rays of both of my wrists (the left suffering more severe damage as I am right-hand dominant, so I had only naturally started sawing my left first, leaving my left hand with less damaging strength to sustain to the right), and a 12 hour abstinence of any food or liquids prior to surgery. As bad as hospital meals are, they at least put some structure in your day. Breakfast, lunch, and dinner, wheeled by a hospital kitchen staff member, greeting you as if you are a guest in a hotel, presenting a tray of inedible and incredulous food ensembles. It is probably as rewarding to some patients as a frozen TV dinner, or Chinese or pizza provided by a strange delivery person at your lonesome home, but as incongruous as it may seem considering my drug and alcohol consumption, I have always exercised a strict discipline with what I eat: food is not a comfort consumption, like drugs and alcohol, but has to be a nutritionally resourceful feast high in protein. An ounce of protein for every pound of muscle just to maintain my physique; more intake of protein to gain volume as well as weight. 200 ounces of protein to maintain a 200-pound muscular body. Not happening in the hospital, where food is cooked in volume with no regard to the loss of nutrients, much less the emphasis on carbohydrates to sedate the sedentary customers.

As I was wheeled into the surgical theater, Dr. Bravados was present to receive me as if I was a guest at his party with a coterie of surgical assistances (maybe 6?) ready to perform the production they had most probably participated in as seasoned stage actors. No time was wasted. I was quickly introduced to the pleasant voice of the anesthesiologist who in less than 60 seconds explained his function and the instructions I was to follow ("count backwards from 10, 9, 8, ...") which after 8, I lost consciousness and any conception of time, much less the invasive invasion to my person on both of my hands, wrists, and forearms. With the exception of my tonsils removed at the tender young age of four, I had never required hospitalization much less surgery. I was a perfect human specimen, not even plagued with vision problems requiring eyewear. Now both of my hands, wrists, and forearms were being sliced open like a pie to expose the object for my surgery, the severed tendons, leaving more stigmatizing scars up my hand and down my wrist then I had inflicted myself.

Up to this point of my life, my preferred drug of choice were stimulants, never interested in losing a moment of my so-called glamorous life to the sensory deprivation of downers. But 6 hours under coma-inducing anesthesia made me reassess my judgement of consciousness depriving suppressants. Physiologically, I was relieved of the excruciating pain I would have experienced had I been conscious during 6 hours of neurosurgery. But it was the carefully timed weaning from the extreme anesthesia when I regained consciousness that gave me one of the most unforgettable and happy drug hallucinations to date. Still under intense surgical lights required for the medical actors to enhance their execution in the surgical theater, I regained consciousness staring up into the uniformly costumed surgical team, Dr. Bravados in the center of my field of vision, the haze of the anesthesia tricking me to think that I was surrounded by a coterie of revelers at a morning party on the beaches of Fire Island, New York. I have many genuine memories of frolicking at dawn on the empty beaches with my disco mates after a long night of drugging and dancing. Fire Island is a gay mecca, unlike any other gay destination on Earth, conveniently located 2 hours from NYC. It is the Disneyland for homosexuals. I felt love for everyone staring down at me in the surgical theater with their masks intact, mistaking these anonymous professionals who had been slaving over my damaged body for fairy tale memories of a time and place far from the immediate circumstances; Fire Island in my golden years during the 1980's. The love I felt could only be expressed with my eyes, and as I became cognizant of the reality of the situation, I continued to dispense the love I felt for the surgical team. Not just for the expertise and time these strangers had devoted to salvage my self-inflicted wounds, but because the anesthesia had produced one of the most ultimate of euphoric highs I had ever experienced. I only wish I could wake up from a night of such pleasant dreams every morning to put a smile on my face. I believe Propofol, the drug administered to Michael Jackson as a sleep aid, is an anesthetic to heavily sedate patients undergoing painful surgery, that lead to the singer's untimely death. It was his salvation as well as his downfall. I know understand why my mother insisted on an epidermal during childbirth. No desire to experience the miracle of childbirth at the price of murderous pain. Just recover consciousness and accept the reward later. Michael Jackson just wanted to escape from the painful reality of his life as a confused overexposed celebrity and an overworked performer. I only wish I could have rescued him from the dangerous support team responsible for his well-being.

The hospital arranged for a Social Service administrator to commence the necessary paperwork for my application to receive Social Security Disability Benefits, as the projected outcome of the best neurosurgeon was not promising for any future employment opportunities, and Medicaid was instantly approved to satisfy the hospital that my 3 week stay amounting to $120,000. would be paid in full, as well as future post-hospital services like in-patient rehabilitation residence, out-patient counseling, physical therapy treatment for my hands, medication, therapy, dental appointments, . . . a load off my mind that I would not bring my parents to bankruptcy, and a newfound respect for the bureaucracy of government after grieving over decades of increasingly unrelatable tax deductions from my ever-increasing paychecks. FICA, or Social Security, was administered as it was designed; an insurance policy for American taxpayers.

I was fitted with matching casts that encompassed the length of my forearm up to my knuckles on both hands, with steel rods to prevent any movement of the wrists to ensure that the reattached tendons would heal over the next two months with no interference of normal functions of the hands. My exposed fingers had 40% nerve sensation, limited to the pinky, the closest side of ring finger, and outer most side of thumbs. I had severed the major tendon, which effected the use of the rest of my fingers and hands.

The Caribbean bodyguards would have to perform all tasks requiring my compromised hands: eating, drinking, urinating, hygiene, and operating MY rented television's remote control. I was granted a Morphine drip post-surgery once I was placed in a hospital room to recover, and remember the heightened sense of euphoria I felt in my otherwise dreary surroundings which I attributed to the Morphine, which was prescribed to alleviate the excruciating pain I would feel building in intensity at the point of surgery, my wrists. As the Morphine drip ran dry and I became painfully aware of how sensitive my damaged wrists were to the slightest sensation not so much from the self-infliction with the butcher knife but from the surgeon's delicate neurosurgery reattaching major tendons as well as the swarms of nerves swimming around the focal point of the operation, I wanted relief. At the first sensation of distress, I politely requested the bodyguard to alert the qualified and authorized medical staff that I needed more Morphine. But as seconds amounted to minutes waiting for the nurse to arrive with another bag of the painkiller to drip into my entire nervous system, the crescendo of pain in my wrists was like sharp jabbing pins multiplying with each second, and my demands for relief evolved from polite to rude. I was desperate for respite from the pain and had no patience for the hospital's response time. I was begging like an addict for more of a medication that I never would have called a drug of choice, but my damaged hands were the vortex of my being under these unusual circumstances.

After a restless week recovering from surgery, I was informed by the resident Psychologist that it was mandatory for me to spend a week in the Psychiatric Ward of the hospital, standard procedure for suicide challengers, to contain the uncertainty of more abusive behavior under supervision in a safe contained environment. , I accepted my fate, but silently resented that I would have to be huddled with people I would still not want to classify myself amongst: "crazy". The psyche ward was referred to as the "Flight Deck", a catch phrase for the mental ward of post-Vietnam V.A. hospitals (usually the top floor) where vets would go to get medication adjustments, escape from the world, drink coffee and smoke incessantly. The catch phrase "Flight Deck" became so popular it spread into street slang for civilian psyche wards. I was personally escorted by Dr. Psychologist with the backup of two male orderlies to enforce the smooth transition of my hospital patient classification from ICU, surgery, recovery, now sentenced as a perpetrator of a violent assault to myself and therefore considered a flight risk. There was a series of secured doors requiring admittance by a wall phone to lock and unlock, like a series of water canals, all the while the hospital staff remained silent, no opportunity to answer questions much less offer compassion in this otherwise anxiety inducing walk of shame.

The ramifications of this procession to the final area that would be the limits of my world for the next week were clear: there was no escaping. Not a notion I had entertained until I had spent one hour in the psyche ward seated in an uncomfortable wooden chair in the nurses' station, the vortex of operations. Aside from a few vital statistic exercises (height, weight, blood pressure, temperature), I was more or less left to absorb and observe my new strange surroundings, and my fellow residents, some of whom were restlessly parading back and forth along the corridor bordering the nurses' station. The co-ed patients were all dressed in identical pale blue stripped hospital issued formless pajama sets to wear both day and night, shuffling relentlessly in both directions in front of the nurses' station, alone, ungroomed, some curiously cognizant of my new presence, others oblivious. They were zombies from "Night of the Living Dead", sniffing out new blood.

After a reality awakening hour squirming in the wooden chair at the nurses station, I was provided with my first psychiatric evaluation and mental disorder diagnosis by an elderly bitter woman wearing a Catholic habit, with no academic credentials, to listen to my story of how I got to this moment in my life, in one hour. For the first time armed with my otherwise smart cognitive skills, I am prescribed a plethora of medication for physiologically pain, anti-depressants which is a standard diagnosis for any suicide casualty, and non-narcotic anti-anxiety pills that I took but never felt an iota of results from, and a non-habit forming but effective sleeping aid. All in one hour under the authority of a nun. I never disputed the plethora of pills I was required to take, but I knew that the medicine was not going to be the solution. I had to be my own solution. No more institutionalization.

I relinquished all personal belongings to a safe, was issued hospital apparel, but allowed to wear my own personal wardrobe that had to meet the staff's criteria of appropriate (no sex appeal, no slogans, no belts or show laces) that my gracious parents provided along with a care package of my personal sundries. I have sensitive skin, and learned what products are necessary to calm my delicate and pampered outer layer of my appearance, some magazines, and a pack of generic menthol cigarettes that somehow slipped by the overworked and undertrained staff required to inspect any material brought inside the controlled environment of the psyche ward. Knowing there was not an opportunity nor an agenda to satisfy smokers who may actually possess this insidious luxury item, I did not do the right thing and turn them over to the negligent staff to be stored in the safe that contained my personal belongings unnecessary in this lock down environment supposedly free of any internal threats to the psyche ward's lawfulness. I was assigned a double room with a mute old man who snored like a were-wolf. I used my charm and professionalism to request a room change once I assimilated with the current psyche ward population to find an agreeable roommate to at least make at least my private domain in this otherwise exposed environment bearable.

Of the 30 patients filling the co-ed beds in the Saint Francis psyche ward, I was quickly able to categorize the population into the "unfocused" and the "focused", of which I was a member of the later. The "unfocused" were seriously disturbed individuals who acted out in the heavily supervised and scrutinized contained ward in attention catching fashion, were generally highly medicated attributing to their volatile nature, were repeat visitors to the psyche ward, some on a yearly basis, and were avoided by me with my duplicitous defense mechanism of denying that I was any better than them. The "focused" were outwardly normal citizens of society, groomed, some actually attractive, with lives including spouses, children, family, friends, and maybe a career outside the penal colony for mental disorder, all of whom were first time inhabitants of a psyche ward, and we all swore to never make the same innocent mistake that placed us there due to no other action than just verbally suggesting suicide at a moment of desperation in the midst of a chaotic personal drama. We "focused" bonded with each other for emotional support surrounded by the stigmatized antics of the truly crazy "unfocused". We were separated every morning during facilitated group therapy so the "focused" could exercise their superior educated cognitive skills to learn and understand how we ended up in the psyche ward, and coping skills to prevent us from ever making the mistake of returning. The "unfocused" were not expected to do much else during group sessions than to play games or express themselves through arts and crafts. There was a shelf of anti-quated low-quality jigsaw puzzles donated to the psyche ward, but never an object of interest much less the undisturbed focus and time required to com-plete a 1000-piece puzzle of some New England landscape. With some of my focused colleagues as my witness, my juvenile hellion rose from the past to inhabit my 46 year old humbled patient in a lock down psyche ward to in-cite me to open all of the individual boxes of neglected jigsaw puzzles, mix-ing up the thousands of cardboard pieces together like a batter, ensuring no one would ever be able to enjoy the satisfaction of completing one of these time-killing activities. Old habits die hard.

The single week projected for me to reside in the psyche ward turned into two as I arrogantly insisted on not allowing the hospital facility to "dump" me in the easy to place rehabilitation center, "Turning Point", located in the same county as the hospital, which had the excessive capacity to provide one hundred residents a bed. But what this local rehab had in quantity it lacked in quality. The demographic was not categorized as "gay-friendly". It was more "thug-friendly", like Rikers' Island. And the theology was likened to a soul breaking boot camp. But it was mandatory in the penal system of drug induced suicide that I attend a 28-day substance abuse rehab immediately upon discharge from the psyche ward. I played my gay sexual orientation as my trump card to remain in the psyche ward until my father, not any of the attending hospital staff, researched and located a small (30 bed) rehab in Guilderland, NY that identified itself as "gay friendly". The name even ap-pealed to me, like "Glitterland", something from the Wizard of Oz. My father was championing my insistence on feeling safe to recover without fear of holding back my sexual orientation. Unfortunately, my insistence to advo-cate where I was going to spend the next 28 days once discharged from the insanity and institutionalization of being imprisoned in the psyche ward required some patience, as the small 30-bed Guilderland Rehabilitation Cen-ter had to put me on a waiting list until a bed was made available. One week is the standard stay for any patient in the psyche ward. But I was there close to two weeks, all because of my entitled sense of control over the future of my mysterious new life after the disco announced, "last call."

CHAPTER 6

One Excruciating Day At A Time

After three weeks of institutionalization at Saint Francis Hospital, I was discharged into the custody of my 70-year-old father as my guardian, responsible for driving me three hours directly from Poughkeepsie to the Guilderland Rehabilitation Center. Finally permitted to exit the medical complex that I was systematically imprisoned from the EMS, ER, ICU, Surgical Theater, and the Psyche Ward, it was a gratifying to breathe fresh air and assimilate with society again. It was as if I had been re-born, only I was resuscitated, and now I was being transported to an orphanage, a 28-day substance abuse rehab, before I could be brought home to my parents, as a 180 pound, 46-year-old man. Unlike the day I was dressed in a pink hand-crafted sweater in 1958, my father had packed suitable street attire from my suitcase of personal belongings recovered from my last place of residence, the remote cabin in Pawling where I had tried to end my life. It felt good to have wardrobe options.

I found gratitude in the smallest things upon exiting the Medical Industrial Complex of Saint Francis Hospital. Smoking a cigarette after 3 weeks of abstinence. I did try to sneak a smoke in the psyche ward with a pack of cigarettes my father had thoughtfully brought in a "care package", was busted and threatened with seriously threatening consequences but charmed my way out of being sentenced to solitary confinement. Eating a healthy meal at a Panera's fast-food franchise after suffering from the tasteless hospital grub that provided none of the nutrition my rigorous high-protein diet dictated most of my adult life was a delight. And the chance to bond with my once estranged father on the car ride, who seemed to be happily mentoring his middle child as if he identified with me. My father was unconditionally supportive at a time I most needed him. No shame. No guilt. No apologies. I broke into a sob during our last private moment together as we rode the single floor elevator up to the living quarters of the Guilderland Rehab after being graciously received by the receptionist at the rehab of choice. It was like I was going to spend a summer away from home at sleep-away camp. Now a 46-year-old in arrested development, having messed up my once successfully plotted life, I was experiencing the first reward of humbling myself, asking for help, and making amends to my estranged father. I was blessed to have had this unanticipated opportunity as my father's health seriously deteriorated over the next 10 years, and I was able to have the closure with this man who up until this moment, was an enigma to me. I was able to have intimate conversations with my father, about his mysterious past that I know he enjoyed articulating as much as I got to finally understand this man, my father, who I was very much a by-product of. He became my champion when I needed him the most.

I was now a resident of supervised sobriety at an upstate rehab of my choice that advertised itself as "gay friendly", to find the only other "out" gay individual in the institution at that time was a staff drug counselor. There is no way to project the demographics of a rehab at any given time. It's the luck of the draw, like when Elizabeth Taylor checked herself into the recently opened Betty Ford Center for substance dependence treatment in 1983, not to be roommates with Angie Dickenson and share some laughs with Rock Hudson in the unglamorous cafeteria. She may have been the only celebrity there at the time, which could explain how she blended into the democratic populace and ended up romancing and marrying her 8th husband, Larry Fortensky, a former construction worker and fellow patient on Miss Taylor's second stay at the Betty Ford Center in 1988. It was important that I identified and was accepted by my peers at an establishment that was not going to permit any gay bullying. I was not deterred from expressing my sexual orientation when I shared in group, as it was an important part of explaining the heavy substance abuse influenced gay culture that I participated in.

It worked in my favor to present myself as a gay man who had spent many nights at exclusive clubs from the time I arrived in New York City in 1976, like Studio 54, that gave cache and complimentary admittance as soon as my pretty young face caught the attention of the oppressive doormen keeping the large crowd out and the desirables in (youth, beauty, celebrity and wealth). New York City embraced alternative lifestyle well before the Stonewall riots, so I always played the handsome 'gay' membership card to my advantage. I also made a menacing first impression on the other residents with casts on both of my arms, leading many to presume I had a violent history. I was flattered but I quickly revealed the ugly nature of my injuries and humbled myself that the glamorous disco days where I learned to make a favorable impression were now a thing of the past. I was being such a prima donna while attending inpatient groups that I was not connecting with my fellow patients. I always had something to contribute to group discussions that alienated me from some of my rehab colleagues who never contributed in the conversation and were getting sick of me monopolizing the discussion. Besides being the only out gay resident, I was also alienated by my drug of choice: Crystal Meth. No one else had any experience with this gay-friendly substance. It was predominately heroin, crack, and alcohol abusers. I was still outspoken in groups, until a strongly worded anonymous note was left in my dorm room accusing me of being a racist. When I complained to the gay counselor that I was being harassed by a fellow patient(s?), I was reminded by my only other gay brother employed at this facility who had made drug counseling his career that I only had to be there 28 days, and he reinforced that this was his job, and that he would probably be in this melodramatic environment for years. So, I was told to tough it out for the relatively short amount of time I was expected to stay in the drama of 30 recovering alcoholics and addicts who may not identify with my so-called glamorous drug culture heritage. The offensive anonymous note was not ignored the administration of the rehab. 29 of my colleagues sat through an hour lecture on the violation of any assassination of character of a fellow client, while I was noticeable absent, receiving a rather unorthodox session confronting my lack of proper and emotional closure to the loss of my last lover, Sharif.

As my 28 days of rehab came to an end, totaling two months of institutionalization, I resisted the rehab's after-care counselor's suggestion of committing to a year of living in the strict structured conditions of one of the many half-way houses in my hometown of Poughkeepsie. I bolstered my case against further institutionalization because I had a safe home to go to, with parents who unconditionally loved me, and were both veterans of 12 step programs themselves: my father was 30 years sober and a member of AA, and my mother a dedicated and huge advocate of Al-Anon. Because I had no legal charges, I was not mandated by the judicial system to commit to more institutionalization after being discharged from rehab. But to have some structure in my belittling experience of living back home with my parents as a middle-aged man in my old bedroom turned into a guest room, I agreed to attend a local outpatient program daily.

After being hospitalized, institutionalized, and rehabilitated for two months, I was discharged to continue living my life of liberty and the pursuit of happiness with no legal restrictions in the safe home of my origin where my retired parents welcomed their troubled middle-aged middle child to feel he was still loved and had a home. No half-way house for me! But suffered severe depression at night as I danced quietly around my retired parents' nocturnal routine. After eating dinner peppered with what I suffered as "small talk", I sat outside staring at the stars smoking cigarettes before retiring to my guest room to read or watch DVDs on my laptop to avoid further social engagement with my elder parents. I needed to escape and live on my own.

Graduates from rehab should have 28 days or more of being clean and sober, which is considered enough time to return to previous established lives, salvage and repair the damage incurred, and abstain from the regular behavior that would lead to another collapse. I was told of old-school bars in downtown Albany, not far from the protective suburban address of Guilderland Rehabilitation Center, that accept the official AA 28-day coin rewarded to graduates in exchange for a gratuitous drink. Recovery is just a cog in the economic wheel of substance abuse; where there are detox and rehabs, there are dealers and bars. It's part of a self-feeding cycle, like life after death.

Some graduates of substance abuse centers, even some otherwise citizens of society free of any criminal record who incur the now dangerously prosperous police activity of trolling for potential suspects of DWI, DUI, DWAI, eagerly throw their souls at the mercy of AA as a cheap ($1.00 donation per meeting) means to beating a jail rap. Some, even I, can dance their way through the AA protocol to achieve the scientifically significant challenge of 90 days of sobriety, when the human body supposedly has detoxed the poison of substance abuse, and the mind has had a chance to neutralize. But each person in sobriety is as unique as each baby born on a given day, sharing a common birthdate for life, but little else. The only consistent instruction bequeathed on a "newbie" to sobriety is to "stay sober and attend AA meetings". I've done that. I've encountered spiritually motivated meetings, usually when I've had the tenacity to raise my hand and speak from the surface of my damaged soul, and I've encountered frustrating confrontations from supposed well-meaning old-timers who want to break my sensitive soul by directing character assassinations that are hurtful and I walk away resentful of that individual's license to tell me such unqualified statements like "Your problem is your Ego" as they physically assault me with a jab to my muscular shoulder blade. I've learned that as much as I've achieved by developing my body as well as my self-will, I can't please everyone, because everyone has issues that have nothing to do with me, and I stick with the people, as I would in a drug-induced disco, who are on the same page as me. I learned that there are basically two types of AA meetings, much like our country's divisive political system. Conservative / fundamentalists and progressives (i.e.: Republic and Democratic). The former, like Catholics, hold meetings comparable to bible study groups, whose members believe and quote from the antiquated origins and intent of the 12 steps and traditions published without revision 80 years ago, like the 10 commandments of the earliest published version of the 'Holy Bible'. These groups, usually unable to articulate for themselves, insist that "if it ain't broke, don't fix it". Being a blue-blood democratic, I sought out and regularly attended more progressive AA meetings, where even the annual International Convention or Alcoholics Anonymous recognizes there is room for contemporary interpretation of the founding principles of AA. Ergo, my proud allegiance to "We the Agnostics", who innocuously node to a chapter in the AA 'Big Book', while allowing the attendees to express their frustration with having to adhere to strict religious protocol while trying to be honest and real with yourself like "turning your life and will over to God", or closing the meeting with the 'Lord's Prayer'. Without categorizing myself as an 'atheist', today's AA is willing to allow me and other unconvinced secular souls living life on life's terms that 'agnostic' is politically correct. But with so few "Agnostic" meetings, I must sometimes "follow the party line" and attend and participate in otherwise conservative old-time AA meetings without rocking the boat, just to feel that I am entitled to my feelings, opinions, and who I consider friend or foe. AA is no different than any other social club.

I attended a local post-rehab aftercare program, where I sat with a mixed bag of drug court mandated pot dealers, alcoholic women in denial of their responsibility to attend substance abuse therapy after driving infractions attributed to the influence of mind-altering substances, and men who were post-rehab, but unlucky enough to have caring, understanding, and support-ive family who would let them return to their homes ever again. I never robbed, much less borrowed money from my parents, but I begrudgingly attended the daily out-patient groups even though I was not mandated by a court of law. The grown men and women, some with spouses and even children, had no option but to live under the strict rules and conditions while residing in half-way houses run like strict boarding schools as opposed to court mandated incarceration in prison.

In addition to intimately meeting with a variety of drug counselors at the outpatient facility I voluntarily attended (I made no qualms about becoming a counselor whore as I requested to change counselors until I found the one who I felt fit my needs), I sat in various themed group sessions that I dis-covered were bearable only if I actively participated by talking a lot. I also saw a bohemian doctor, whose job it was to prescribe meds for my disorders, both clinically diagnosed and self-professed conditions. Unlike most text book doctors who just wanted to hasten the time spent with a patient, this unusually personal doctor was much more interested in my daily interests, activities, and nutrition (my lifestyle) then the standard "have you entertained suicidal thoughts" at the start of each of our sessions. He took me off Prozac to replace the old-school anti-depressant with the popular X-generation mood enhancer Wellbutrin, like a good strong shot of caffeine, not knowing that Wellbutrin was the very medication I mistakenly overdosed in an attempt to kill myself. He also told me I needed to inject some carbohydrates in my otherwise protein-centric diet to alleviate the anxiety I was already not happy was becoming my outstanding daily struggle. Anxiety, invading my dreams, would produce heart palpitations upon first waking up, thinking about my past transgressions, and what looked like a hopeless future that would always haunt me, tempting me to consume alcohol to temporarily ease the discomfort. This bohemian progressive doctor was also employed to treat inmates in prisons, and I liked his prescription to medicine as an experiment for each of his patients as unique individuals, never assuming one size fits all with his diagnosis and cocktails of meds.

I was also in the unexpected position of qualifying and obtaining the approval of a handsome monthly revenue courtesy of a distant cousin I had never met, the Social Security Disability benefits program. For the 25 years I worked in corporate posts, I never thought much of the FICA deduction on each paycheck, other than the fact that after totaling all the deductions on progressively bountiful paychecks, I was only receiving approximately 60% of my gross income (?). Once broke and unemployable, it was explained to me that because I had been working corporate jobs from 1981 -2002, with paychecks diminished 30% by F.I.C.A. contributions, a rainy-day future that I never included into my life plan. The money from SSD was much more than I could have fathomed, but I was assured that the revenue was all money I thought I'd never see again.

My last paychecks as a consultant brought my insane salary over $100,000 the final year of my corporate career. This was my money, I was not a charity cause, and this benefit and program was meant to become available should I become unable to work. I was dumbfounded as if I did not deserve this generous windfall. But because I had an excellent paper trail documenting my physical and mental conditions from all the professionals I engaged with since the advent of my disability (read: suicide attempt), Social Security was gladly and responsibly willing to pay for all my medical treatments by endowing me with a carte blanche Medicaid card. That was in addition to my monthly tax-free benefits check that put me in the lower-middle class income level. Never in my wildest dreams would I have expected this unexpected windfall, and would gladly sat at a table in a high school on career day advocating the importance of getting a legitimate job that was paid "on the books", so that one day Social Security, as it was designed to do, would be there for you. I was approved within two months of applying for Social Security benefits without a lawyer representing me, and was treated with the upmost respect by the interviewing Social Security agents who left me in disbelief after I was told the amount of my monthly income I would receive that would allow me to exist comfortably on my own, without having to work. The Social Security agent assured me that this is exactly what the program (the FICA deductions) was designed for: I had been contributing to an insurance policy for a rainy day like the one I was currently drenched from, and the large salary I garnered as a consultant in my successful adult professional the last few years of my career had filled the coffers of my Social Security benefits; this was not a government handout. This was my money, put aside for a rainy day. Now it was pouring.

I needed to get out of my parents' safe house, not only because I felt my presence was not fair to their retirement after they had fulfilled their obligation of raising three children with the goal of sending each of us off to college and a life independent their guardianship, but I was also uncomfortable having built a prosperous life as an adult (I had owned and flipped for profit three pieces of property) to find me with no other option but to be the son that had nowhere else to go. It had only been two months living with my parents, but I could not see the gratitude in it, couldn't humble my arrogant self, and with my first Social Security check, inflated by including previously qualified benefits that accrued until I was officially approved.

I secured a great apartment in the most exclusive residence in the upstate city of my origin, like I was living in an exclusive uptown Manhattan high-rise. I had never lost the sense of entitlement to deserve the best. Easily able to make the monthly rent and buy new furniture and grocery shop for my-self, I was also able to commute to local AA meetings and make shopping trips riding on public buses without owning a car. I felt like Mary Richards, leaving the humble bohemian studio in Phyllis Lindstrom's Victorian boarding house, leaving the intrusive landlord and brassy neighbor Rhoda Morgenstern after promotions at WJM studios to afford and award herself the contemporary high-rise apartment in a luxury building with a views of one of the ocean-like Great Lakes. It was identical to the Chicago high-rise used as the stock footage in the introduction to the "the Bob Newhart" show, exemplifying an American ideal reflection of a successful urban professional; work hard, live well. I lived in a well maintained, secure, doormen high-rise with beautiful terraced views, and an enormous clover leaf swimming pool where I could perform skilled swim laps in my body confident Speedo, an unusual choice of bathing attire for someone my age and in a conservative community that expects men wear to wear knee length boxers. I like to tan, and a Speedo allows me to tan my legs, producing a sexy brief tan line that I admired in the privacy of my picture window size bathroom mirror. Swimming laps, emerging from the pool with inflated muscles, and drying my water soaked body on the pool side lounge chairs to soak up the energy boasting rays of the sun to the delight of many lonely housebound widows watching from their apartment windows, and a surprisingly large percentage of gay male residents, gave me the validation my exhibitionist narcissism still thrived on.

I graduated from the outpatient program after six months of what I successfully portrayed was unfailing sobriety to my coterie of medical and mental health professionals who treated me. In truth, there were many undisclosed relapses out of boredom with my "new lease on life", but was not willing to talk about the details of each one of these relapses like promiscuous sexual liaisons, as I knew the particular circumstances of each alcoholic episode was of no interest other than he singular fact that I wanted to change the way I felt with readily available substances rather than confront the demonic feelings that I felt only alcohol could appease.

My first task upon returning to civilization was to enlist myself as a soldier of Alcoholics Anonymous to battle the forces of evil (drugs and alcohol) one day at a time, by attending the ever-available AA meetings held every day at practically every house of worship. My hometown of Poughkeepsie had changed from high-tech IBM-land to drug infested Recovery-land, with an abundance of AA meetings, half-way houses, outpatient programs, and Detox centers to combat the drug and alcohol culture that had blossomed in the now economically depressed City of Poughkeepsie.

I would arrive minutes before an hour-long AA meeting to minimize the amount of my life I was willing to invest in staying clean and sober. Meetings would either stimulate me or stifle me about my membership in this archaic albeit the only successful 'tried and true' non-profit organization keeping alcoholics sober for over 80 years. It was suggested that I volunteer my services to give back what I had so selfishly taken from society living as an alcoholic drug addict, and AA would humble even the most entitled ass by providing service commitments at these so-called egalitarian meetings. Setting up chairs, making coffee, post meeting kitchen cleanup, and taking outreach speaking commitments to other AA fellowships both near and far were comparable to court mandated community service. I liked to spend as little time at an AA meeting as possible, so none of these demeaning service agreements agreed with me. I offered my advanced skills as a state licensed fitness trainer pro-bono to staff the gym a few hours every week at a YMCA located a short walk from my plush urban digs. I was still carless. Volunteering in early recovery was a means to repent for past unbridled hedonism. It was a cake job at the local YMCA, with duties as limited as monitoring activities of the members in the gym for ten unpaid hours a week. It was such a relaxed, unsupervised atmosphere that I got away with sneaking a good slow workout for myself while still fulfilling my duty of monitoring the gym facilities and its patron.

It wasn't long before my ego and my greed recaptured me to negotiate with the Y's management for a salary on par with my illustrious fitness work history and skills reflected in my resume and my perfectly sculpted physique. The fact that I possessed a valuable state fitness certification also boded well for the YMCA's credentials. I felt a better motivator than selflessness to perform the human services job for this community-based organization was a regular paycheck. My entitled way of thinking had returned after only a few months since my devastatingly self-indulgent attempt at self-annihilation, leaving both of my hands permanently disabled, entitling me to an impressive Social Security Disability Income to sponsor a comfortable employment free lifestyle. But I was working in a gym, instructing clients on how to properly use the equipment, and I myself was lift weights to strength train, albeit with some added focus and adjustment to my previous regime due to my inability to grasp any bar on a dumbbell or cable machine securely or for more than a few seconds. If I had been spied on by a Social Security agent, I would have some explaining to do.

I actually got sober (a couple or false starts, until before I knew it, I had a solid year of genuine sobriety) and was offered part time salaried employment at the YMCA, careful not to endanger my Social Security Benefits by working below the allotted quota of monthly income. My next goal was to buy a car. I wanted to fulfill my childhood fantasy of driving a muscle car. Not a responsible decision, but a reward to the concessions I made living in unglamorous Poughkeepsie. So, I bought a 1969 Chevy Nova that needed a lot of work not by me, with two disabled hands and not mechanically inclined, but by a dedicated and supportive mechanic one block from my apartment, ironically "in the program". The benefits of having been a member of the AA fraternity. The Nova took a lot of money (credit cards) to restore, but it gave me the satisfaction of fulfilling a dream as well as garner the attention of many men impressed with the car, which fulfilled the unrequited validation I still desired from men, even though they were heterosexual and interested in the car and not me. I had put my homosexual desire to lay with a living, breathing, satisfying man after I left NYC back in the closet of sexual suppression. Porn was more manageable.

My prized Chevy Nova was spared the elements of severe weather and theft safely ensconced in the high-rise's underground parking garage. I had five years clean and sober, discovered more progressive AA meetings and sober colleagues who I could relate and not compare with in the neighboring, more progressive college town of New Paltz, in Ulster County, after a long high speed trip in my muscle car restored from a jalopy to a show car quality that made me proud to drive every day in town. Public transportation was exclusively for the unfortunate carless population that I was once a humble member of, and my disciplined and narcissistic attitude about my appearance and health that bolstered my ability to appeal to young and old, not to mention distracting from the fact that I was a very 'out and proud' homosexual, even though I was no longer a practicing one. I was well aware that I was living in a not so progressive county that whispered to me to not push my personal sexual orientation while still advocating for acceptance in the new social world of the young adult generation I mentored, and a job that impressed those who interacted with me (family, new friends, and my employers) that I could not simply behave as a narcissist, a role I had learned to perfect while living in NYC. I had a job that relieved me of the obsessive compulsion to focus on how I appeared and how I was interpreted by the rest of society by taking the focus off myself every day in lieu of caring for another member of the human race, at least for the fifteen hours I was paid to perform each week. The YMCA deserved my attention, and I deserved to devote myself to improving the lives of young adults.

After about 5 years of monthly visits to a community based mental health facility, I was no longer willing to continue receiving group or individual therapy because I did not see any reward from the medication nor the public service therapists. Also, as I parked my enviable 1969 Nova muscle car in the parking lot and passed the indigent clientele loitering outside the entrance waiting for local low-quality medical cab service, and the claustrophobic waiting room where I discreetly avoided eye contact with my peers to avoid any social interaction or identification, I did not have the disposable income to seek more acceptable treatment and more effective medication, so I made the executive decision to quit, including discontinuing the meds I had been regular taking 'cold turkey'. Even my mother warned me of the dangers of not even weaning myself from psychotropic medication that I may not believe was working, but after immediate discontinuation, I felt empowered until I didn't. Once life threw me some shit, the shit hit the fan. I could not cope. The meds, as innocuous as I found them to be, were like Social Security; contribute now for the insurance to recover when a disaster occurs.

I followed the dictate from rehab that there is actual recovery from drug and alcohol addiction by regularly attending AA meetings ruled by the tenants of their fundamentalist 12 step program to change behavior or substance abuse obsession. AA was the only option available without a generous health insurance plan. I resented this life sentence, felt like I had to become a convert to the dependence on Jesus Christ and God as my only salvation, but made the most of it by finding a home group where I liked the vibe of the members, implemented alternative AA activities to interact with others in recovery on weekly softball and volleyball games using my ambitious resources to secure permission from the Parks Department and the YMCA to host these events at no cost. Non-competitive and co-ed, it was my way of saying that there are alternative ways for recovering alcoholics and addicts to feel the sense of community that AA strives for but have some sober fun without sitting through a structured AA meeting. It was also my way of breaking the stale mold of AA that I was always at odds with. I took a long half hour ride over the river and into another county to attend a weekly agonistic AA meeting in the town of New Paltz that was more progressive with lifestyle choices, and the agnostic AA meeting in a neighboring county that gave me the respite from the more fundamental meetings that I was lim-ited to in the conservative county I lived in. I took speaking commitments representing my home group, would prepare what I was going to say, but if AA instilled anything in me it was the ability to get over my fear of public speaking. I found that as long as I talked candidly about my experience, I had none of the nervousness I suffered from standing in front of a classroom of my school peers trying to enlighten them about a science project that I had plagiarized and did not fully understand myself. If you really know the subject you are speaking about, like your own real-life experiences, it's un-complicated to talk to a large audience of strangers.

So, I went to 3, then 2, then 1 meeting a week, was responsible showing up early for the weekly softball/volleyball events, as I was accountable for the use the fields/courts. And then I got an opportunity to work with home-less youth, which as much as it made me feel I was providing a role model to the clients, reminding them that I had to learn to avoid the very mistakes young adults, like I once was, are prone to. I was slipping on my dedication to my own recovery. I had once been told by a drug and alcohol counselor who understood I did not exactly enjoy sitting through AA meetings, that because this counselor, who was clean and sober, was devoting her career and time helping struggling alcoholics and addicts, she did not deem it ne-cessary to attend AA meetings at the end of a long day at her job. That notion stuck in my head like an old wife's tale; I was expending all my energy helping those in need, so by the end of the day, I was too emotionally exhausted to participate in what I came to see AA meetings as a mind fuck. I felt that at the end of the day, I had done the right thing and helped another individual which is the remedy to getting out of my sometimes sick and dangerous head, and believed that I had beaten the desire to ever drink without reli-giously attending AA meetings that felt like a life sentence to obsess over the recover/relapse/recover reality of alcoholism.

I was a reward-oriented smoker, maybe 5 cigarettes a day, using the mind-fulness technique to enjoy the nicotine consumption undistracted from any other activity (driving, phone calls, watching a movie at home on DVD), and an elitist attitude by becoming a member of the "organically grown", socially conscious, and hard to find consumer of "American Spirits" cigarettes. I developed a cough that would wake me up, which I would attend to by keeping a bottle of water by my bed to soothe my irritated throat. Eventually, my grocery list included cough syrup (no alcohol) to keep handy during these nocturnal coughing jags. What I discovered by accident was a way to get high from consuming a larger than recommended dose of the syrupy liquid cough suppressor, thinking I was not violating one of the most important principles of being a member of AA: the cough syrup label indicated that it was free of alcohol, so, I went on buying more, drinking more, and getting addicted to drinking cough syrup all day, functioning on it to drive to the gym to work out, go to my job requiring me to be tenacious to target areas in our county that had high levels of disadvantaged teens likely to run away, and be responsible to mentor teens who accompanied me on these trips where I was the responsible adult driving the company vehicle, public speaking engagements to audiences of students and professionals, while sipping a tonic I had prepared at home consisting of cough syrup, seltzer water, and pre-workout powder, Creatine, which was empowered with extremely high levels amount of caffeine extract. Nobody, my buddies at the gym, neighbors in my nosey apartment building, my co-workers, family, friends, or the professionals I was required to meet with in academic settings seemed to sense that I was slightly invigorated by the ingredients in my omnipresent "tonic" water. I was once approached by a club owner who had been informed by a concerned and noisy patron who had observed my innocent public display of supplementing my bar bought seltzer water ordered with a bouquet of fresh fruit bar condiments with a small vial that contained the powdered creatine that I was perhaps concocting a "roofie" for myself and my alcoholically impaired date, only to make the whole ridiculously innocent explanation, and my entitled status at the club as a colleague of the party promoter or DJ. I felt shameful when I had to present my ID to prove I was over the legal age to purchase, in my case, as many as 10 bottles of cough syrup in one visit to my local grocery store. It was open 24 hours, so I would feel less shame about purchasing copious amounts of cough syrup afterhours.

I was attending private house parties that all the other revelers were energized by alcohol and cocaine while I was able to avoid the party's vices. What I was doing, drinking cough syrup, was to my surprise not a unique proclivity but was quite common amongst ambitious (mostly teens legally too young to buy alcohol) given the street name "Robo-ing". After looking

"Robo" up on the internet, I found that my secret "tonic" that stimulated me through my long day and into the night was as close to the high I felt when I had carefully calculated crystal meth with alcohol. The only difference, in my mind, was that I was not surreptitiously buying meth from a paranoid drug dealer, and I was not purchasing alcohol from the forbidden and skanky liquor stores that I still took note of but blotted from my mind as not part of my custom. Robitussin brand cough syrup had become a new part of the young adult vernacular for those who wanted to get high over the counter by "Robo-ing". And it was my latest drug of choice.

I was living well (nice apartment, impressive restored vintage muscle car, a job that made me feel I could make a difference to the world), yet I was addicted to my cough syrup-based tonics to keep me functioning day to day. I was a veteran of the black-market designer drugs NYC dealers were selling to me to enhance the escape from reality that the dance clubs in NYC promised and delivered. And here I was thinking I was over that lifestyle that almost killed me in NYC, convinced I was no longer a drug or alcohol abuser, and I could not enjoy a moment of my waking day, work a respectable job in non-profit, or socialize with what little nightlife upstate New York had to offer without my robo-tonic. A few of my non-judgmental friends (active drinkers and users) thought it was a bit weird that I stuck with this drug of choice, but I had a good run with it, never having any consequences legally or medically. I had read up on celebrities "robo-ing" until requiring hospitalization for seizures, but the only medical condition that started disturbing my normal lifestyle was explosive diarrhea, which woke me up with a gurgling stomach warning me to dash for the toilet, where I would remain for 10 minutes violently emptying loose bowels, contemplating the health of my internal organs, and disturb my ability to fall back to sleep. I wrote my first book in three record months which I attribute to the enhanced connection the cough syrup facilitated to the period music I played while relapsing into my memory banks of how great these classic Disco hits conjured the emotions and feelings that allowed me to tell my story: *Homo GoGo Man: A Fairytale About A Boy Who Grew Up In Discoland*. Every moment of my life could be rejuvenated by a song from my romanticized past. After two years of daily consumption of cough syrup, the euphoria the medicinal liquid initially gave me turned on me, leaving me experiencing dark, suicidal depression. Being a stubborn alcoholic, I would not learn my lesson that what was once my drug of choice was now poison, and the insidious insanity of not ever learning that which is no good for me would still find its way into my system, bringing on darker and desperate misery.

I had a good run with the cough syrup. Almost two years without any bad experiences besides the explosive bowel movements in the middle of the night. One of my confidants made me think about the cost of my over-the-counter habit. Buying generic instead of the real McCoy Robitussin, finishing 3 bottles ($6.00 each) on a normal day (if I were to go out at night I'd need more), I was spending close to $600.00 a month. I don't think crack addicts can justify such a monthly expense. But I was addicted, couldn't go through a day without it, and still believed I wasn't violating my sobriety.

CHAPTER 7
Employable RX Addict

Now that I was paid to perform at the YMCA, my old ambition to excel reignited in me to implement innovative youth fitness programs that new scientific research indicated was not harmful but beneficial for not yet fully developed youths to engage in when exercised carefully. I arrogantly sold these research findings to impress the management of the archaic YMCA, as well as the parents of my new fitness students during a meet-and-greet orientation. I was ambitiously climbing out of the humble hole of where my indulgent lifestyle had taken me: the bottoming out of life where tomorrow doesn't matter. I was a maverick introducing young YMCA members how to utilize the fitness equipment, an area that was once exclusively for adults, to become skilled at concepts and routines that would hopefully become part of their exercise programs for the rest of their lives. Like a practiced ballet instructor, I would reinforce the importance of good form to prevent injury, as well as instruct them on proper gym etiquette that I knew was overheard by the old dinosaurs that had populated the YMCA less as a fitness center and more as a social setting. I knew their tin ears were tuned into my youth fitness diatribe, surreptitiously teaching the old dogs new tricks.

Through all my years of excessive self-indulgent unhealthy behavior, I maintained regular attendance at a gym to perform intense strength training to balance out healthy physical activity with the destructive lifestyle I lead outside of the gym. I was also obsessed with gracefully maintaining my sex appeal as the decades separated me in age from the new flesh on the competitive beauty contest of the club circuit. My philosophy of working out spills over from sexy body to positive self-esteem as well as grace in all other components of life, like navigating through a crowded dance floor to find the perfect spot to feel undistracted and free of dancers who lacked the natural dance rhythm I possessed. I am a dance floor narcissist. The gym has always been my temple of worship. I thrived on mentoring my young pupils at the YMCA, presenting the façade of a role model that had skeletons rattling inside my perfect exterior of muscular armor.

Six months into my convenient, low pressure, esteem and fitness building job at the YMCA, I had reaffirmed my confidence that I could still mentor young adults on how to avoid the pitfalls of my own life experiences that I had set me on a course to drive head on into an irreparable crash and burn. I wore long sleeves while I trained my young clients and when interfacing with their parents to disguise the violent scars on my wrist indicating I was not exactly the role model they were entrusting with their impressionable and inquisitive offspring.

The historic YMCA was actually in the town that I grew up in, where I was enrolled as a junior member in a Saturday afternoon program, and left by parents to spend the entirety of the day utilizing the athletic facilities: the pool and the gymnasium, playing volleyball, basketball, soccer, dodge ball, and a game room with pool tables, air hockey, and assorted boring board games as well as impossible to complete puzzles because of missing pieces. I already admitted to being responsible for sabotaging the jigsaw puzzles at the Saint Francis psyche ward.

Without warning to the staff or the members, the YMCA closed its doors due to poor finances three months into my employment. After a year of neglecting to pay the electric bill, the non-profit facility's power was cut off, presumably without notice. It was a shock and embarrassment to members and staff to realize the YMCA facility, like a bad theater production, had "gone dark". This YMCA had been practicing a benevolent business model focusing on being more than a revenue generating membership-driven gym by persevering its presence and dedication to providing free youth services to the local financially disadvantaged community. Today's existing YMCA organization is now a strictly 'for profit' business, focusing on membership contracts that excludes any 'Christian' brotherhood values. Thank 'Planet Fitness' for turning the fitness industry from a seriously effective but expensive endeavor to change people's health and physiques to a budget conscious social club.

But I gracefully bounced back from this otherwise unfortunate loss of a productive job that provided structure to my day and money in my wallet. I was blessed to be immediately recommended for employment at a prominent local non-profit organization dedicated to homelessness. With my reputation and success advocating for young adult programs at the YMCA, I was confidently hired to work for a division of the non-profit homeless organization, specifically to address the unique and sensitive needs of the young adults "at risk" of homelessness. I was offered the "luxury" job of outreach coordinator. I made appointments to network with other local organizations servicing the youth of the county, as well scouted locations where homeless youth would populate, reaching out to this otherwise disposable general population that had little clout to prevent them from unfairly being removed from their dysfunctional homes and placed in the discouraging foster care system and/or probably run away, encountering dangerously exploitive situations and a bleak hope for a healthy life affirming future. I was welcomed into a team of sincerely caring professionals who wanted to save the world. This non-profit wanted to make a difference in the still hopeful lives of our young clients who had experienced very difficult childhoods due to bad parenting and unsecure homes. My public relations job was to bring awareness to the issues specific to the young adult homelessness epidemic. The job required the finesse of networking with existing organizations and professionals targeting the same population, most of which had better finances (i.e.: Planned Parenthood) who I would dovetail strategies with to create events that would attract and interest the otherwise "system wary" clients, and establish trust and rapport with the disadvantaged youth that I encountered by relating to their hard-luck experiences with some of my very own reckless experiences. I may have been articulate, well-groomed, educated, driving a brand-new company car always full of gas to traverse extensive miles around the enormity of Dutchess County, but I always let a client know I was no better than them. I, too, was an occasional teen runaway from my suburb home, albeit never for more than a single night and fortunately consequence free. Driving a new fuel-efficient KIA Soul company car for hundreds of miles a day around our large diverse county of jurisdiction was a real perk considering my primary means of transportation was an inappropriate 1969 Chevy Nova given its age and uneconomical gas consumption. I bought the Nova as a jalopy to drive locally, and with the help of a lot of credit cards renovated to the status of an eye-catching muscle car of my childhood "Hot Wheels" dreams. I felt entitled driving this unpractical choice of primary means of transportation, as if I was still reveling in my troubled adolescents and the risky lifestyle, I had fallen prey to, survived and progressed from. I got off on the attention the car got, as if the car and driver were a source of envy to the "everyman" who were resolved to drive generic automobiles. My vintage Nova Muscle car was an extension of my personality. And while my impressionable young clients at the homeless shelter admired me for this flashy ton of debt I insisted on driving daily and maintaining monthly year round for 10 years, I always told these hopeful young adults that I had many opportunities to mess up my life, and that if they wanted to have the life/car/job/apartment of their dreams like me, they could. Mentoring is so much easier than being a parent. The responsibility stops when your shift is up.

I had forgone therapy, psychotropic medication, and my affiliation with AA when I ingenuously learned of the severe cutbacks in the budget to non-profit youth programs in our state, as mandated by the New York State Governor's office, and being a "luxury" item employee, I was told my job would be eliminated. I was no longer medicated, which left me responding to this life crisis intensely; close to a nervous breakdown. But because of the good relationship I built and maintained with the parent organization of the youth homeless program, I was offered a transfer of employment to work in the agency's overnight emergency adult shelter. It was the only adult homeless shelter in the entire county, ironically housed in an ancient and long vacated dormitory that once housed the certified insane. Night after night, my fellow co-workers and I were required to enforce tough crowd control measures to contain the desperate adult homeless who would show up at a designated location in the city to hopefully get checked in for a guaranteed bed, or turned away for drunkenness, drug addled, outstanding police activity status, or "bad" behavior on a prior stay at the shelter. There were physical riots and emotional breakdowns from hopeful homeless guests who had spent the day wandering the streets, felt entitled to the beds, meals, showers, transportation, counseling and mentoring that the shelter generously promised them, 365 nights a year, but were rejected for various reasons. There were regular guests at the shelter who never seemed to make an effort to see their daily nomadic existence as temporary, and I could see how life on the streets hardened most of our clients. Talking with them individually, they did not see any way out but to take the free service offered to them by this non-profit agency as if it were an unalienable right. I no longer could use my old skill set that worked for teachable young adults who still had a chance and hope for a better life. I could listen, sympathize, but could not offer any comprehensible advice. I was now herding desperate, drunk, stoned, drug-addled and bitter homeless adults who I was dumbfounded did not find me relatable, simply because I was not homeless, drove an enviable muscle car, was in great physical shape, polite, articulate, even patronizing to get everyone to behave and get along. It was only after a few weeks working in this new territory of homelessness that I hardened as well, realizing that the ever-returning homeless adult clients did not respect my good manners and judicious decisions, but would try to take advantage of me. Or worse, mock me. I was reduced to reinforce the duplicitous attitude of my fellow, tired, bitter, long-term colleagues, who, with no proper education, training or skills, fell into this job, and found that even if their personal lives were not much morally better than the homeless clients, they could employ the privileges of the job's authority while in this thankless vocation. There was a distinct division of citizenship in the shelter, with the clients generously provided a clean bed in the only local adult shelter, like in a prison, and the staff, professionally untrained to perform population control. We were no better than them, except we had a salaried job to pay our rent where we slept without the hardships of a homeless shelter inundated with rules enforced to expel a client. It was an oppressive environment with specific strict mandates enforced by the staff (me) which made us the enemy to our clients. The staff were given the title of 'property managers', with the sole goal of preserving peace, but we were more like wardens in a jail. I began to resent the clients.

I started the job with an optimistic attitude, but between the never ending conflicts with belligerent, drug-addled, alcoholic, mentally ill clients, and the lack of proper training and qualifications of my co-workers (who hated their jobs), each evening shift at work turned into a nightmare where I found myself being disrespected by clients (nothing personal) and apathetic management that did not care to bend rules to make the shelter and staff appear less tyrannical and more humanitarian.

I was clean and sober 8 years at this point. I did not qualify my two-year run consuming cough syrup as a violation of my sobriety. I was in alcoholic denial. But I experienced so many uncivilized conflicts with clients and staff at the adult homeless shelter that I romanticized how alcohol could bookend a bad night on the job. I was sober enough to play the tape and remember my past personal experiences and the serious consequences of the poisonous effect alcohol had on me. But I was confident with 8 years of abstinence from alcohol and drugs, bolstered by attending a progressive recovery group of what I felt were my intellectual peers gathering for a legitimate but threatening offshoot of the 12 step program called "We the Agnostics" on Sunday nights in the serenity of the town of New Paltz.

I felt I had beaten the AA proverb of "the desire to drink". However, on my new job with a new client base befittingly housed in an abandoned insane asylum, I became aware that the legal pharmaceutical meds that my clients, who had no jobs, no homes, and no caring families, were luxuriously supplied by doctors with an abundance of strong (read: narcotic) meds sponsored by the almighty powerful Medicaid card. These health care professionals that treated the homeless by generously prescribing heavy doses of powerfully mind-altering meds knowing that Medicaid, the gold card of medical services for the economically disadvantaged, would generously pay for the 'top shelf' drug (not generic when cost is not an issue) was shocking to me given the clients' life circumstances. Homeless, unemployed, drunk and drug-addled clients refilled their meds each month at little or no cost. The meds were a very marketable commodity. The homeless and jobless client saw these meds as a cash cow to their otherwise poverty level situation. The Doctors' diagnosis and prescription for a disturbing physiological or psychological condition was not of importance to the client. The shelter client would rather sell their prescription then follow the doctor's orders to take as instructed.

Never mind that the prescribing Doctor felt these were necessary daily supplements to their client's otherwise aimless lives, these quality meds were easy money to a population that were willing to forgo the powerful effects of these anti-anxiety, pain-killing, attention deficit disorder, sleep deprivation, and more serious psychological diagnosis medications (Lithium!) by selling them at a mark-up from the pittance they paid to a drug inclined human like myself. And I worked as an employee to monitor them. It was unethical, but unavoidable.

I had recreationally ingested substances deemed illegal and dangerous to the human condition for decades as the norm within the NYC club and drug culture I thrived in for 25 years. I had a history of consuming alcohol and drugs at a rate that was not socially acceptable. After "bottoming out" and recovering, for 8 years I was legitimately prescribed psychotropic medication by medical professionals that knew my history and framed my life in basic models of mental illness categories: addiction, alcoholism, depression, suicidal. And all the non-narcotic medication that the pharmacological professionals kept tweaking for my mental welfare never made me feel any different, better, or secure. They all felt like placebos granted to me to think I should feel good when in fact I thought they were all a big waste of my time. I complained of the low-level anxiety plaguing me from dawn to dusk for 8 years. Not any of the cocktails of anti-depressants or non-narcotic anti-anxiety meds eliminated the semi-regular occurrence of a low level panic attack, usually occurring in the early morning near sunrise, as I would be wrestling with some anxiety themed nightmare of some reoccurring experience in my past, and my conscious mind would bail out of resolving in dream state by waking me up before my designated or desired time to rise and shine and start a new day. Starting the day with dreadful panic attacks seemed to be my penance. Once sober, I relished bedtime as a time to escape from the realities of life, but it was never pleasant dreams. And being woken by a panic attack and not being able to fall back to sleep irritated me as I wrestled with the bed sheets and the demons in my unconsciousness that woke me. I would find myself starting the day with a very uncomfortable level of anxiety that I would fantasize could be cured only by early morning alcohol consumption, an activity I was familiar with to smooth out a night of consuming sleep deprivation drugs. But none of the mental health professionals would take my anxiety complaints as seriously as I wanted them to. I was classified as a drug addict, so all effective anti-anxiety medications were off-limits.

So of course I didn't think that accepting a single unfamiliar pill from a compassionate shelter client who could see I was a bit stressed, or because I had gone out of my way to appease a shelter guest by bending the rules, as a violation of my 'sobriety'. I would quiz the donor to tell me what it was that I was eagerly willing to swallow with positive results to my state of mind that were immediately appreciated. Klonopin, Xanax, Valium, Oxycodone, Percocet. The otherwise stressful stint working at the shelter was smoothed out by the pill. I was in euphoria and happy to accommodate almost any demand from the high-maintenance clients. I saw no infraction with my 8 years of sobriety. It was secret, a gray area of what I still defined as being clean and sober. I was as duplicitous as Courtney Love acting out in public apparently intoxicated, yet insisting she is clean. As long as I wasn't drinking or drugging my substances of choice, I was still able to convince myself and the world who knew me that I was still clean and sober. On prescriptive medication illegally shared with me, I was functioning and didn't seem to suffer any side-effects. I soon engaged in illegal transactions with shelter clients who were now by definition my 'drug dealers'. They were gifts. They help elevate my stature amongst the clients at the shelter from an enforcer of authority to a trusting confidant. Soon it was common knowledge that I could be culled into favors with the tip of a narcotic med. I discovered that most of my co-workers were highly medicated individuals themselves who felt they could not perform their compassionate duties on this stressful, unpredictable and potentially dangerous job without the help of mood altering meds, some legally prescribed, some acquired from acquaintances who were happy to exchange a full vial of narcotics prescribed for some aliment, but didn't care to take. I guess some people really didn't want or need what was prescribed to them, and that's the difference between an addict and a person willing to live with a serious mental and physical condition without their Doctor's respective prescribed medication. On a job responsible for the welfare of homeless adults granted a safe place to eat, shower and sleep instead of a surviving a night on the streets, I inadvertently found access to the very drugs that my own health care professionals were depriving me of. I was finally enjoying the relief of my anxiety and the stress of working and living without the option of alcohol or illicit drugs in a historic asylum now serving as a homeless shelter. I had unlimited access to Xanax, Klonopin, Valium and then the boost of Adderall; all of which made me feel better than I all the psychotropic meds that had been prescribed to me and had taken regularly for 8 years, and that I wanted to believe would make me forget about all the illicit drugs and alcohol I relied on for 30 years of my adult life to produce that false sense of happiness I thrived for because what I now was ingesting were pharmaceutical, legally manufactured and distributed in this medically obsessed country. I was very chemically happy. I felt love for the pharmaceutical drugs that I was acquiring second hand from the medical industrial complex. No side effects, no hangovers, no impatient waiting room visits to get prescriptions for medicine that didn't bring me the euphoria I was always reaching for at any cost. I was living in a fool's paradise with a trap door I couldn't or wouldn't see.

After an ugly dispute with an ugly coworker acting as an ugly supervisor, I filed a formal complaint with the human resources department of this otherwise civilized homelessness organization. It didn't take a lot of tenacity to proceed with this formal action as I was well versed in the requirements of any business to ensure that every employee had the right and duty to report any unjust behavior witnessed by co-workers. It is whistleblowing, but it is also cathartic to have a human resource administrator perform their job of protecting the image of the organization and avoid potentially lethal legal action. I was granted my day in court presenting my case that the job environment at the adult shelter was in need of reform, my candor and opinions were respected, but unfortunately the adult shelter and the way it was run was not a priority of attention to the sinking ship of this once generously funded and prestigious non-profit homelessness organization. What felt like was a winning meeting with the highest levels of management of the organization was actually a defeat when I was again informed of what I was deaf to: the private and public funding that allowed this organization to prosper, keep well paid but unmanageable employees happy, was focusing on a new business model of making ambitious forays into the prosperous future of real estate investment. The shelter would continue to run as it had for years, regardless of the dismal lack of positive results to the hopeless and growing homelessness locally and nationwide. I was too smart to keep the status quo of the unattractive adult emergency shelter program, and even with the bump of gifted meds, I could not dummy down to perform this insensible job.

I submitted a lengthy resignation, giving gratitude and acknowledgement to the organization for allowing me, with a sordid history I revealed during my exit interview, to avoid future backlash and arouse emotional support for my ambition to prosper. But I spelled out all the infractions I witnessed and inappropriate behavior I had personally experienced on the job, but that document was more cathartic than effective to my proactive decision to leave the toxic environment than to effect any healthy changes to the otherwise low expectations of running a homeless shelter in an abandoned insane asylum.

"Carlos and Carmen Vidal just had a child

a lovely girl with a crooked smile

Now they gotta split 'cause the Bronx aint't fit

For a girl to grow up in

Let's find a place they say, somewhere far away

With no Backs, no Jews, and no Gays"

"There but for the Grace of God Go I" by Machine 1977

CHAPTER 8

Black Market Rx a Pill A Day Keeps the Doctors Away

I left the insanity of striving to provide some semblance of order to the lawless atmosphere that characterized the adult "emergency" shelter I had been begrudgingly employed at for four months, with access to pharmaceutical meds from the clients I was responsible for supervising. The plethora of pills got me through the unpredictable night shift at the insane asylum/homeless shelter before I decided to resign from the unempowering job. However, my drug addict mentality gracefully accumulated contacts to maintain black market access to the meds I was now accustomed to, naively developing into a narcotic addiction, which allowed me to justify the unethical action as an means to acclimate my mental welfare now free of the insanity at the shelter. When I was no longer employed at the facility, I was now a convert to the miracle of modern medicine offering a solution to the day to day stress and strife of life; narcotics. All the non-narcotic meds I had been legitimately prescribed to take regularly for depression, anxiety and sleep disorder by a licensed nurse practitioner for the past 14 years were bogus. I had now acquired a taste for the altering meds that effectively elevated the class of my mental health, most of which were narcotic. Once, I was a NYC "drug of the moment" disco bunny, buying and taking one dose of illicit recreational mood-altering substances at a time. I was a now a prescription pill popping junkie, with vials of precious pills at my disposal to take not as prescribed but as I desired, depleting my supply before I could rationally project. My body and mind did not like it when I could not supply them with latest narcotic drug of choice. I experienced acute Jonesing.

I had acquired the phone number of a particular client at the shelter, John, who received an ample monthly supply of Adderall and Klonopin, medicine a licensed doctor had determined John needed to consume daily to provide a crutch for the mental illnesses he was diagnosed with: Adderall to address his attention deficit disorder buffered by an anti-anxiety med, Klonopin, to smooth out the peaks of the Adderall stimulant, preventing insufferable panic attacks. John was more than happy to sell a good portion of his monthly supply of both meds to me for the financial windfall that helped supplement his negligible subsidized income of food stamps and Social Security Supplemental Income, at the expense of the pharmaceutical treatment of his mental health. John was a sweet man, who had a soft spot for me as a role model, slightly homo-bro. I believe what cemented the deal of his aggressively offering his prescriptive medicine for sale personally to me was that he was trading his one marketable asset, his pharmaceutical medicine, to procure alcohol and crack, his preferred drugs of choice.

Our relationship developed from client/staff to dealer/addict intimacy one particularly tumultuous night while I was still working for the shelter. I was enforcing the protocol of that non-profit institution that professed to address the issues of the growing adult homeless population in addition to providing emergency shelter. John was one of the 100 regular homeless adults seeking shelter with our organization seven nights a week. On a poignant winter night, a particularly heavy snowstorm was escalating into a dangerous blizzard that no human without proper shelter could have survived. At the appointed hour of 6:00pm, the shelter staff had arrived at the inner-city check-in location to register the desperate homeless crowd to the full capacity of the 100 shelter beds with complimentary bath and meals. The second phase of the operation was the tedious job of packing and transporting the guests from the check-in spot in the center of the city to the converted 'asylum-cum-shelter' 10 miles away in a secluded wooded hill on the outskirts of the city. It took multiple trips to transport the 100 clients with limitations on carry-on bags with only two passenger vans, a task that required the staff to exercise crowd control and optimism over the hour it took to traffic 100 human beings from the check-in location to the shelter. It took at least an hour of multiple roundtrips for the two commercial vans to complete the human transport. I was assigned the lonely task of supervising the anxious crowd at the check-in point, outdoors, in the same inhumane freezing conditions as the homeless, to ensure the registered clients maintain some semblance of order. I was to babysit the homeless adults like school children during recess, monitoring and reporting any illicit activity: smoking pot, drinking, fighting, health failure, and leaving the property of the waiting area to procure or indulge in any of the above transgressions which was grounds for me to reject their coveted guarantee of a bed at the shelter. I was not strict in enforcing the shelter's protocol for client behavior, but I did exercise my authority where I saw violence, bullying, disrespect to property, inappropriate and out of control behavior, which would put me in a precarious position protecting my physical as well as my emotional welfare. I was working alone, so I had to make my own executive decisions on how to handle situations. I welcomed a peaceful, uneventful night gracefully interacting with the clients, establishing relations, making suggestions, and insight some hope, as I had also experienced homelessness and the consequences of that experience in my life.

John had arrived at the shelter check-in late that foreboding night, missing the mandatory registration to guarantee a bed in the warm shelter that 100 other homeless adults were counting on to survive the night's blizzard. As the jitney of vans transporting that night's guests were shuttling back and forth, I was left behind outdoors in the blizzard representing the only member of the shelter staff, keeping some semblance of order to those homeless adults anxious for a ride in the overcrowded vans to the warmth and safety of the historic asylum tucked remotely on a wooded hill. As I tried to keep myself from freezing in the cresting snow storm while keeping the anxious clients waiting in the same inhuman weather conditions, my primary purpose was to intercept any physical and verbal conflicts that would inevitably erupt, a peace keeper with no backup or special equipment other than my own cell phone to call 911. A lot of the waiting clients would break the shelter's rule of abstaining from alcohol and drugs to medicate and entertain themselves. They knew I was aware, but I was not going to begrudge the waiting clients what was second nature to them; self-medicate with a staff member who would not interfere.

John showed up post-check-in (approximately 6:30pm) clearly intoxicated, cause for him to be denied a bed at the shelter in addition to being late. I took a bold and aggressive action to ensure John's welfare on this desperately dangerous night when he direly needed shelter from the storm. I was performing my duty of ensuring that a homeless human being would not die from hypothermia, very possibly suicide, if not an overdose from medication to escape the agony of feeling hopeless. I knew the acting authority on all activities at the shelter as an emotionally unstable man who had no authority over any of the staff, but, had a vindictive personality disorder that would flip from openhandedly silly to prickly dictator. When I first started working at the shelter, I slowly scouted out my boundaries with my colleagues before developing trust and confidence as backup to my authority on the job, but the titular boss I knew I would have to play the charm card to neutralize the possibility of a power struggle considering his long-term employment at the shelter facility, and my fragile position of "last one in is first one to go". I knew he would be threatened by my presence as an obviously overqualified and over educated co-worker who could be seen as a challenge: emotionally, physically, and spiritually. There is an assumption that all gay men are in alliance under whatever circumstances, but the truth is that gay men are as more obsessed with social hierarchy than demonstrated in less advanced species of the animal kingdom. Both he and I were gay, but from very different perspectives. I saw the transfer of assignment by the non-profit homeless organization from young adult "Outreach Coordinator" to adult emergency shelter "Property Manager" as a demotion in stature, even though I retained my executive level salary (a secret I had to keep from my new shelter co-workers). As much as I approached the administration with alternative jobs with my experience and expertise to advance the cause of the organization (I had a degree and experience in writing effective policy proposals), I was stuck with the undesirable night shift job of 'property manager' at the shelter to maintain the hopeless cycle of adult homelessness infecting the bucolic county I lived in. I took some snarky remarks from my so-called boss (again, he had no authority over me, as much as he tried), and even reported inappropriate conversations my fellow homosexual colleague made the mistake of uttering while on the job, to no avail with the Human Resources and Administration. They saw the offensive unprofessional employee as someone who would do the undesirable job without complaining or leaving. The emergency adult homeless shelter was not a priority to this non-profit organization. They were cognizant of my gay nemesis' ethical, moral, verbal, and physical violations, but calculated that no one else on this Earth would perform this thankless job except him, who had no scruples.

The night of the deadly blizzard I was standing with 50 anxious homeless adults freezing in the seriously frightening storm conditions waiting for transportation to the shelter, with no other colleague as backup, when John showed up physically incapacitated from intoxication, over medicated, and emotionally weak. He knew he was not entitled to a bed at the shelter due to his tardiness, made all the more pathetic as he knew he was responsible for his predicament due to his own self-indulgent illness. John, an adult in his 20's, began pleading, crying, and sobbing to me to provide him shelter, or he said he was sure to die. This was not a private conversation. I had 50 anxious and freezing homeless adults waiting for a van to transport them to the shelter, watching and waiting to see the outcome of one of their own. I was outnumbered 50 to 1. There but for the Grace of God, go I.

I followed protocol and called my so-called boss who was safely protected from the outside elements in his warm office, but in his usual chaotic mode of insisting on controlling everyone and everything in what he perceived to be his kingdom, and without consideration or discussion with me about the circumstances I was in, barked his verdict about providing emergency shelter to John, giving me the directive to call the Police to take responsibility for John's situation off of the ogre executive's hands. He hung up without so much as concern for my precarious situation: a mob of 50 homeless adults already bitter with any representative of authority in their lawless lives watching to see how the newest staff member, me, was going to function in this drama, outdoors in severe blizzard conditions.

I did not call 911 as instructed. I asked some of my supportive, and yes, drug catering clients to surround John with assurance and physical comfort as I called the home phone of the director of the emergency homeless shelter, a woman I always kept an excellent professional as well as personal rapport with throughout my employment at the non-profit. I apologized for the intrusion to her private life at home after her regular work hours but explained my predicament. Without the need for more than the informative sentences that my professional experience taught me as the most effective form of communication, the director immediately agreed that the situation should be resolved in the compassionate manner our non-profit would insist as a mantra: no human should be denied shelter, especially during a deadly snow storm, and she would overrule my vindictive faux boss. I won my case (I am quite good at manipulating a situation to my advantage as an insidious alcoholic and drug addict), and the audience of 50 freezing clients agreeably acknowledged my heroism. John was now crying and hugging me out of relief, and I had now stabbed a fellow gay co-worker in the back. One of the sweetest and popular regular clients knew I was concerned by the wraith I was to face upon finally returning to the shelter to be confronted by my nemesis, the gay co-worker whose authority I had undermined by calling his boss to ensure John shelter that night, and she provided me with an un-known sedative to buffer the predicable confrontation.

When I finally packed the last bag of belongings of one of our homeless clients into the last jitney van and sat in the front passenger seat contem-plating the defense I would deliver to the projected confrontation with the co-worker I had undermined, I kept my conversation to myself. There was no need to rally the support of the clients who had witnessed the incident, as they were clients, and this was a matter involving two staff members of a non-profit organization. The moment I arrived at the shelter, my nemesis called me into a private office to blast me for my insubordination of his dictate to turn John away and threatened me with the guilt that his job was now in jeopardy. But I knew I had made the right decision, and just like the wicked witch threatening Dorothy wearing her dead sister's ruby red slippers in Oz, I was able to laugh at my psychotic co-worker's rant by reciting the line of Glenda, the good witch: "Be gone, you have no powers here".

John was forever grateful that I did what any human being would have done under the circumstances, but he truly would always see me as his hero, and I now had a personal drug connection to his monthly Medicaid provided medicine of Adderall and Klonopin.

Shortly after I resigned from my job at the shelter, John began receiving Social Security benefits to secure a rental apartment, ensuring he would not have to seek shelter at my previous place of employment, and he began working in the restaurant industry where he found he had the skills and talent to excel in a respectable and marketable career in food preparation. He even expressed interest in committing to further his education in this competitive but lucrative profession. On the day John was scheduled to begin working in the kitchen of a highly successful restaurant/catering hall overlooking the scenic Hudson River, a promising opportunity he deserved, I committed myself to ensure he would be driven to his new job by me, with the added incentive of acquiring more of my now new drug of choice: Klonopin. However, the morning he was expected to report to his new job, he was found dead, presumably from an overdose from a lethal mix of drugs and alcohol, at the age of 28 (?). I will never know if his death was intentional or accidental, as I was worried about the authorities discovering and questioning my association with John. He was a friend, but he was also my now deceased dealer.

CHAPTER 9

Dr. RxXnX

"Doctor Love, he can kill my every pain,
He can make me well again.
Doctor Love, he ain't got no competition, he writes my prescription."
'Doctor Love' performed by First Choice (1977)

At 52, I was now an historical substance abuser; 20 isolated adult years of benign recreational illicit drug use evolving to chronic substance abuse, sprinkled with 15 years of incongruent abstinence that may have classified my sobriety as schizophrenic. During the periods of my life that I was honestly clean and sober, I categorizing my lifestyle as "in recovery" when offered and graciously refusing the social wheel greasers of alcohol and cocaine from my nocturnal friends as I resisted the AA caution avoiding "People, Places, and Things". I went to AA meetings at 7 pm. But come 11 pm, infused with the vibrations from my personal disco collection playing on my bass heavy surround sound system, my high-end wardrobe, the mirrors I used to expand the dimensions of my studio apartment which were akin to the multi-mirrored hallways of the Palace of Versailles in France, my loneliness of never meeting a salacious suiter who hadn't already transplanted his fine ass to NYC began to make me desperate for gay companionship with boundaries. I began associating an outrageous clique of Poughkeepsie partyers, not deterred by their open substance use at parties, clubs, and bars out of desperation for glamorous company while living as a fugitive of NYC. I had already slipped into the "grey area" of pharmaceutical abuse, which resulted in my suffering from severe anxiety disorder on a semi-regular basis when I was devoid of my narcotic drug of choice, benzos. It was debilitating. I would wake in the luxuriously appointed comfort of my apartment in Poughkeepsie to an uninvited and physically torturous panic attack which I could not wrestle away under the covers of my bed. I would surrender to the assault on my sleep and sacrifice the serenity of my Posture-pedic mattress and matching pillows, the sun rising on my eastern exposure picture window blocked by my floor to ceiling Levolor vertical blinds to keep my apartment nocturnally dark. Sleep was important to me, ergo the bedding and blinds. I would not categorize my sleep obsession as an indication of depression. A minimum of 8 hours of sleep has always been part of my devotion to the muscle recovery necessary from my intense weight training. I was in denial that drugs had finally conquered and successfully enslaved me to their consecration.

But woken by an anxiety themed dream that would raise my heart rate to an uncomfortable and frightening level resigned me to shorten my quota of sleep, forcing me to start an unwanted day earlier than I desired. With John gone, I no longer had access to the meds that I felt improved the quality of my life (Xanax, Klonopin, Valium), so I started drinking again. Vodka. First thing in the morning. Daily. If there were not a few shots left in the previous day's bottle in the freezer, I would get anxious and drive my muscle car in a tunnel vision similar to those I experienced on drug runs to quench my overwhelming need for alcohol. It's like sitting behind the wheel of a self-driving car; I could operate the car and follow the rules of the road without incident, but subconsciously, as all my alcoholic or drug obsessed mind could process was obtaining my drug or alcohol. Self-conscious to the point of paranoia that the world would recognize my insidious alcoholic obsession, made all the more intense as I drove my attention attracting muscle car to various local liquor stores, sometimes forced to wait in empty parking lots in a humiliated and uncomfortable state until the store would open at 9:00am. I'd dash in discreetly, grab my Vodka, pay with some charm to somehow think I was disguising my obvious alcohol disorder, dash to my prized car in the still empty parking lot to open the bottle and swig the burning liquid until I was ready to drive home in some improved degree of comfort. This went on with my family's knowledge and some of my fellow alcoholic neighbors' delight for 3 months, daily, after 8 years of abstinence from alcohol. Alcoholics keep company with other alcoholics. So, I always had company to offset the depression of getting drunk alone. Especially needy alcoholic neighbors with no jobs who wouldn't care what time or day of the week it was; as long as there was fresh booze offered by another generous alcoholic who had already conquered the sober quest of driving to a liquor store.

My family traditionally celebrated my birthday, my father's birthday, and Mother's Day together as one event at the family home each May with many of the diverse kinsfolk that now represented our contemporary family. The year I turned 57, I was told by my sober father that I was not to attend the event under the influence of alcohol. I never kept my drinking a secret, and would bring my Vodka to the family house for dinners grilled on the large modern gas-fueled barbecue my parents were so fond and skilled at using that it was utilized year round requiring multiple trips up and down a flight of stairs to cook and return to the kitchen or dining room deliciously grilled chicken, salmon and steaks. So being my told by my father the condition to my appearance at my own birthday party, probably to spare my young nieces what could be interpreted as "unacceptable" behavior, I was a bit resentful, but respected his request. However, as the day of the event evolved, I felt a more uncomfortably anxiousness about the family affair as the clock continued its relentless march to 6:00pm, the estimated time of my arrival. I could not and would not show up with alcohol on my breath, but I desperately needed some relief, so I bought two bottles of an old companion that use to be my drug of choice until I had to say goodbye years earlier: non-alcoholic cough syrup. My extended family was preparing for a multi- kinfolk celebration. My boyfriend, Storm, was by my restless side as I moaned and groaned projecting an eminent disaster. Two bottles of cough syrup finished by 4pm, and I was reminded why I stopped "robo-ing". I did not feel euphoric, or socially functional, as when I had started my once newfound drug of choice, cough syrup, that fueled my existence for 2 full years. That's why it was at one time my drug of choice: it did not seem to interfere with my ability to work, socialize, eat, sleep, etc. But in this instance, I was reminded why I desisted from consuming any more cough syrup; recreationally as well as medicinally. My fun run was over, and the thick substance became poisonous to my mind and my body. Two hours before Storm and I were expected sober at my family home, I was physically incapacitated from this desperate relapse, leaving me paralyzed in bed, where I made what I thought was a mature decision to call my family home to report that I was in no condition to drive, and would have to cancel my attendance at my own birthday party, most disappointing to my pre-adolescent nieces visiting from Buffalo to see their cool "Uncle" Chris and his loveable partner Storm. My mother accepted my news with no comment, as if I was the best judge of the situation, but I could detect the discontent. She was an excellent product of 30 years in Al-Anon. She could detach from the alcoholic in her life. But I could still sense her clenched teeth over the 30 second phone call. I told her it was not alcohol, but cough syrup that made me incapable of driving to the family event, as if that would absolve me of some remorse. I promised I would make an appearance the following morning after sleeping off the cough syrup overdose. That would be the very last time I would drink cough syrup. I advocate against the consumption of the insidious over the counter medicinal remedy to friends and family who complain of disturbing coughs from winter colds.

The next morning, I called the family house to announce that I was ready to drive my BF Storm in my muscle car to the family house for breakfast and any events I missed the previous night regarding the two birthdays and Mother's Day. My sister, a Gemini who wavered from soul mate to alter ego, answered the phone with a stern directive for me to stay put, do not come to the family house, and an ominous warning that she would be over to my apartment shortly with her partner, a no nonsense hugely successful attorney. I sensed my freedom was in danger, as my sister and her partner can make me feel like a criminal with their serious lesbian / parental / financially successful stance on life that made me feel like the frivolous infantile unattached family fag, until Storm and I became life partners in 2013, becoming my plus-one at all future family gatherings, raising my stature and self-respect as a more mature member of our diverse family. Storm was seen as the grounding influence on my otherwise reckless history of boyfriends. It's as if I was now a more legitimate member of society by committing to a life of quiet domestic bliss that made me more relatable than when I was known for nothing other than my devotion to disco parties.

My intuition and guilt were projecting an ugly state of affairs, not a friendly 'gay siblings with partners' brunch. I quickly rushed my BF Storm out of the impending situation by taking him to the train station. I was alone and ready for the jury of my sister and her partner in my well-appointed home to hear them out.

But I was not prepared for the precision of their verdict: In my absence the previous evening, my family had performed a modern day witch hunt called an intervention, concluding that I, an independent adult, needed to be mandated to detention in a medical detox facility, and they had already arranged for me to be admitted to the very same local hospital that I ironically found myself institutionalized in 2004, Saint Francis Hospital, which happened to be equipped with a fully operational detox clinic, with a clause that attendees of the detox would be transferred to the institutional rehab in the same hospital after successfully detoxed. This was the very same hospital I was transported to by the EMS team 9 years ago, where I was institutionalized for a whole month before discharged to the comparable civility of Guilderland Rehab. The hospital rehab that was associated with the detox I was booked by my family to attend was none other than the ghetto rehab I had dodged a bullet not sent to by default after my psyche ward stay in 2004; the overcrowded (100 beds) Riker's Island of rehabs for thugs who had burnt bridges with their own family, leaving them with no options. It was like a cruel episode of the Twilight Episode. Deja Vu only relocated to make sure I would not ignore the call of the demon rehab back to haunt me.

I was not consulted if this was what I felt I needed or wanted, and what plans I would need to address or alter while institutionalized over the next 5 weeks. I had a life, responsibilities, bills, and multiple situations that I needed to personally address, none of which I was willing to postpone for 30 plus days with no warning or preparation. Then there was the fact that no discussion transpired acknowledging that I had no medical insurance for said services, leading me to believe that my tough love family mentors, who literally have lived their life with no financial restrictions to cheat them of their perfect dream life of luxurious and spontaneous acquisition of material possessions, never once broached the subject of the incurring medical bill I foolishly assumed they were generously willing to paying for. After all, booking me into a detox might have included a discussion initiated by the medical facility as to the payment method (i.e.: insurance). Everyone in my family who unanimously voted "detox Chris" knew my financial and insurance situation but seemed to overlook any discussion of this matter in my absence. All they seemed to be obsessed with was incarcerating me for bailing out of a family gathering. I at least deserved a proxy vote.

As strong willed as I always was about managing my existence, I did not resist my sister and her legal partner in their interference and manipulation of my independent life, and so agreed to go to the detox when they bluntly announced this drastic upheaval to my independent adult life. I was given no say in the matter. I had been to a substance abuse rehabilitation center ten years earlier, so I knew the drill: pack a bag of the toiletries I relied on to maintain my healthy exterior, as well as all prescribed medication. One small shoulder bag. No change of wardrobe. I was being rushed by my hostile unsolicited visitors on an early sunny Sunday morning day from my birthday with their own agenda. My plan was to appease the family by entering the detox facility peacefully, and then use my charming will power and first-hand experience to make the visit short so I could return to my home and resume the freedom of living my life independent of any family or authority. After all, the rent and bills were paid by me. None of these financial responsibilities were given attention.

I had left my car parked on the street that dreadful morning after rushing my BF to the train station to spare him the ensuing family theatrics. As much as Storm adores my family, his loyalty is to me, and he did not argue or question my rush to discharge him. He understood that I was at least exercising what little actions I needed to enact as an adult trying to practice some damage control before relinquishing my right to campaign for my life before the powerhouse couple of my far from alcohol-free sister and her vice-free life partner joined in wedlock who seemed to make clear that they were taking control of my life. Now that I was a single entity prepared to advocate for myself, I explained to my responding family wardens who declined to visit me in my apartment, but mandated that I was to come to them outside my building by their luxury car; their jurisdiction, not mine, giving them a position of power. Once it was understood what their intentions were, a ride in the back seat of their car like I was under arrest to be taken to the detox, I sensibly explained that I would need to move my car that I had hastily left on the street, instead of in my paid and reserved indoor garage space to avoid any traffic parking violations. Innocent and logical to me but interpreted by my suspicious interlopers as a possible attempt to escape from my impending sentence of institutionalization. I presented my plan to move my car as perfectly reasonable, but the act itself was embarrassingly silly as they kept a small space cushion between our respective automobiles as I performed my duty of placing my car in the safety of its reserved garage space. My chaperones were prepared for an impulsive car chase out of a crime drama TV movie. Point one for me. I was not giving them the satisfaction of putting up a fight. I've heard of interventions that have resulted in deadly, violent, unforgiveable conclusions when opposing forces go to war (families, the law, vengeful engagements, greed, retribution, …), so I suppose my family was projecting and protecting all parties from an ugly outcome, but I not only did not want to cause any more harm to my family's all so important reputation, but I also knew I could navigate my way out of unwanted and in my opinion unnecessary futile medical remedies to a situation I knew I could resolve without misunderstanding the players: i.e.: my family. My sister was struggling with her own alcoholism, effecting her relationship with her partner and her children, so her cold hearted actions that day qualified her as a hypocrite. My sister-in-law lived her life like the world was a courtroom that she excelled in. My brother lived insidiously with his alcoholism by denying it, hiding out in cheap hotels to drink in isolation. My father, forced to get sober by his lifetime employer, IBM, gave up on AA and abstained from alcohol for 30 years, dying with unresolved issues. The only guardian angel in my life was my unconditionally loving partner, Storm, who would give me the hope and belief that I was intrinsically doing my best, that he still considered me and my accomplishments super heroic, and he prayed for me while I could not.

While the unconditional love of my life was on the two-plus hour return trip to his home in Jamaica, Queens on the Hudson-Harlem Line of a Metro North Railroad, my mandated ride in the back seat of my sister and sister-in-law's luxury car was only 5 minutes to the Saint Francis Hospital detox ward. Even though there were three of us family members in the car, the silence was long and deafening. I wanted to discuss what was not happening, about ANYTHING, but my female wards were stone silent. It annoyed me to be treated like I had no say in the matter. I felt like an unwanted rescue dog confused about being returned to the kennel. An admissions nurse interacted with my business-like sister-in-law upon our arrival at the detox, a gruff introduction honed by her years in the legal profession. I was not even given any recognition by the intake nurse other than instructed to take a seat, and as much as I expected some emotional intercourse with my sister, the waiting room television provided the only distraction. It was insulting to be ignored by family members who were fulfilling what they silently must have felt was a family obligation to come to my aid by institutionalizing me for my own good, but every time I turned to look at them for some kind of recognition to my state of mind (total confusion and hopelessness brewing into panic), I was competing and ignored by one of the 1000's of syndicated episodes of "Law and Order" that America had made as routine as "I Love Lucy" marathons in my childhood broadcast from the waiting room television.

Upon intake, I conceded to the hospital staff that I had no medical insurance, imagining this bombshell hospital visit to be a generous gift from my prosperous chaperones, but found that once I was trafficked to the detox, I was my own. My sister and her partner gave me a formal and insincere hug and left me to fend for myself, financially and emotionally. I was the middle child, experienced at taking care of myself. Goodbye and good riddance to my fantasy of a supportive family.

My shoulder bag was searched by a security guard, removing my wallet, cell phone and keys that were locked in a safe, leaving me with my personal toiletries (I was not going to rely on institutional soap to irritate my sensitive skin) and my own meds, which were not dispensed to me, but locked in the detox ward safe while the hospital provided facsimiles billed at an disproportionate markup.

I was given a brief interview with a compassionate employee who had no credentials other than her own experience as a recovered substance abuser. Amongst the general lifestyle questions, I kept asking if I could expect some anti-anxiety medicine to alleviate the discomfort I was paralyzed by, a by-product of acute alcohol withdrawal combined with the shock of this breaking news event on the week of my birthday; I was being incarcerated in a detox against my will. I was eventually given a low dose (1mg?) of Valium and taken to my private room on the detox ward. I asked for another Valium every 3 hours, standard protocol on the detox ward, but the mild tranquilizer never gave me the relief I so desperately wanted. I was suffering from acute alcohol withdrawal after a 3-month bender consuming a liter of Vodka a day. The only medical attention I received was a nurse who visited every 3 hours to take my vitals. Even during the night as I slept, the nurse proclaimed his presence by turning on the blinding overhead fluorescent lights, announcing it was time for the regularly scheduled checkup of my vital signs, as if I my health were going to decline and I would eventually be declared dead. He would spend 10 minutes taking my blood pressure, temperature, and pulse rate, while I lay in a stupor having been woken from my deep REM sleep. I never was visited or invited to interact with a health professional besides the residing nurses to discuss what the detox's or my course of action was. After 12 hours of feeling like a prisoner on the detox ward, avoiding the snarky existing residents who seemed like they had been there long enough to have formed a clique that I had no interest investing any of my time invading, I carefully approached the night shift supervisor who did not seem too busy to allow me an unscheduled visit in his office to engage in a conversation about my situation. So far, the only structure in my residence on the detox ward was regularly scheduled vital checkups and an administered valium. Meals were made available in a compact lounge, but I had no appetite. I was determined to manipulate my way out of the detox ward to return to the comfort of my own apartment that was stocked with my own food, not to mention a large silver bowl of my famous red potato salad garnished with chopped hard boiled eggs, dill, scallions, and raw sliced Kirby cucumbers that I intended to bring to the family gathering twenty hours ago. The night supervisor graciously listened to my recovery history, my successful periods of extended abstinence attending AA, my contributions to service to the organization by personally implementing and managing a successful sober softball and volleyball weekly event for five years, how I got hoodwinked by my underhanded family to deposit me in the detox ward, what kind of life I wanted to get back to outside the detox ward (daily attendance and active participation in AA meetings that I already was very familiar with), and this agreeable man received me as honest and sincere, instantly making the promise and executive decision that I should be discharged the next day. I'm sure the fact that I reinforced the fact that I was without medical insurance to pay for the exorbitant cost of my minimal presence in the hospital was a determining factor to arrange for my timely discharge. But like any winning verdict, there was a condition to my vindication; I had to refuse the regularly served Valium for the next 12 hours, and then I could go home.

I was discharged at noon the next day, 24 hours upon my outrageous admission, my personal belongings returned, recovering my own badass gear I favored to present a tough exterior upon first impression, but capable of conveying a genuine exterior of sincerity and gratitude, now that the emasculating backless hospital housedress I was hopelessly relegated to wear on the detox ward was replaced with my cuffed Levi's jeans, Harley-Davidson motorcycle boots and matching belt with a chain attaching it to my wallet, my armor of muscles enhanced with a tight fitting V-neck T-shirt, and an application of hair balm to style my otherwise unkempt hospital bed head. I had to inform the detox staff that they had possession of my own meds locked in their safe, which I expected to leave with, which caused a commotion and delay, but fortified my self-will. It was as if I was holding up a bank. That there was not even a policy to ensure that a detox intake who proactively came prepared with their own prescription of meds were absconded with no discharge protocol to return said medication. My impression of the Detox is that it was not given any serious attention to its function other than to keep a patient in unstructured environment requiring the patient and staff to do nothing more than kill time as they count the minutes, hours, days, and possibly weeks since their last substance use. Valium was the recipe for survival, not therapy or any form of organized activity. But once again, I was advocating for myself, reinforcing that I did not need to be supervised by authority figures to subsist each day "in my shoes" (in my case, my preference for boots).

Once I was expelled from the hospital by the non-plussed security guard, I called a cab from my cell phone as I caught up on my 24 hour abstinence from smoking a cigarette, to return to my very own home, furnished to my satisfaction, and my beloved sound system and music to personify the disco classic " Last Night a DJ Saved My Life". I had called my BF Storm the hellish and lonesome first night at the detox ward on a resident wall phone to tell him how forlorn I was at the onset of the mysterious reality that I was incarcerated in a ridiculously useless institution, and again later that night after I had my successful "day in court" (actually more like "night court") with the agreeable facility administrator. Once I was safely in the comfort of my welcoming home, crudely dug into the bowl of my famous and table-presentable potato salad after fasting for the last traumatic 24 hours, I called my parents' home to inform them of my whereabouts, reaching my "dry drunk" father, who was not rallying to my enthusiasm much less supportive of my decision to check myself out of detox , but instead the old gruff grief and disapproval I was familiar with all of my life as his son. My family expected my detox stay to last a week, at which point I would be transferred to the hospital's associate ghetto rehab run with tough love for society's unwanted, with no outdoor privileges, for another 28 days of my precious and limited life. I told my father that he had no say in the matter, and hung up, disappointed, but once again, motivated to prove to my father, my family, and the world that I could take care of myself, and preceded to make phone calls to reengage my important life.

Once I had masterminded my return to the free world, I was determined enough not to drink that I begrudgingly drove myself to one of my least favorite but conveniently located and regularly scheduled AA meetings the very day I freed myself from the detox. I did not want to skip a beat to declare my third campaign to live clean and sober. I always preferred to drive myself in solitude to and from such AA meetings rather than ask for or offer another member a ride for my selfish mental welfare, to avoid small talk that I would preserve for making my voice heard in the course of the structured one-hour AA meeting, and knowing my car was waiting for me in the parking lot, discreetly leave after the meeting was officially ended (holding hands in a circle to recite a prayer is anguish to my morality, but I begrudgingly do it while performing my own personal meditation to supersede the childish group daisy chain of mindlessly reciting some AA or Christian incantation). Arriving minutes before the start of an AA meeting, making so discreet acknowledgements to my fellow attendees, preserving a calm demeaner during the proceedings, raising my hand to unload the contents of my disgruntled mind in early recovery with no trepidation, staying through the hour meeting to the very end of what can sometimes feel like is the most excruciating hour of my life, make limited if no polite small talk, and beeline for my car where I can turn on my disco music to fill my head with some guaranteed euphoria as a reward for the exercise I just endured, knowing it was for a good cause. My sober serenity.

Sober, over and done with the bureaucracy, cost, and time it took to continue obtaining the legal prescription medications that I truly wished but was disappointed could not treat any of my troubling states of mind (read: mental disorder), I made the executive decision to acquire Xanax legitimately, relying on the referral of one of my soul mates I was blessed to acquire at the foggy start of my recovery 10 years ago. Angie and I would have made the perfect couple, except that we did not share the same sexual orientation. We both liked to validate the male species by their handsome factor, appreciated a beautiful penis, and both thought very substantially of our own exceptional desirability, placing sexuality a high priority in our world, like some people put religion. Angie was savvy enough to ensure that Xanax prescriptions were and always would be a part of her life. I had no hesitation asking Angie to make the otherwise unaccustomed referral to her personal Doctor so I could acquire the medicine, Xanax, that she so loyally lived with. I wanted to feel legitimately treated for my acute anxiety with no reservations, like Angie.

The benign doctor Angie referred me to be a basic internal medicine health professional who held office hours in Mount Kisco, New York, an hour drive from my home. With the introduction from Angie, Dr. RxXnX was willing to see me without going into extensive medical / mental / substance abuse history. Angie had already prepped me on how to successfully present myself as an everyday citizen of society who did not have any problems with substance abuse, a record of public knowledge to any health care professional. I was just going to a sympathetic Doctor to complain of a recently developed crisis of anxiety without explicitly requesting Xanax. The Doctor was an old-school small talker, so I engaged with him on a superficial level all the while anticipating the visit to conclude, a paper script for legitimate Xanax prescribed to me, the CVS pharmacy a few blocks away who was not familiar with me but very familiar with the local Dr.RxXnX to erase any paranoia my guilty imagination was trying to project to ruin this farce, and my moment of reward when I got into my car to open the freshly filled vial of my drug of choice: Xanax, and swallowed a few, disregarding the prescription instructions. Dr. RxXnX would cautiously prescribe me a one-month supply, no renewals, requiring me to make an appointment no sooner than 28 days, to repeat the same stage performance.

I developed an addiction to Xanax quickly, and with my predilection to always seek an altered state of euphoria, I had increased my body's daily requirement of the narcotic tranquilizer, resulting in periods of insufferable severe withdrawal when my monthly allotment was kaput. I compared these days of withdrawal from benzos to those I associated with what I only heard was experienced by heroin addicts. For the 25 years I took illicit drugs while clubbing in NYC, I never suffered from such severe detox. And now I was living a quiet life in the Hudson Valley, but I was severely addicted to Xanax. Physiologically and psychologically. A catch-22 as my drug choice; a love / hate relationship. Xanax washed away the trauma that produced physiologically debilitating panic attacks with no apparent side effects, like alcohol hangovers! Only I never experienced my body developing such an addiction to such a benign substance.

On further investigation, advocating for myself when the psychiatric community followed an obvious protocol signified by their routine standard questions to classify my mental welfare. The physiological discomfort I regularly experienced would lead my polluted cognitive thinking to respond in a unhealthy manner, guiding me to make an emergency choice of action to relieve the discomfort (a panic attack is paralyzing): take more of the legally prescribed Xanax, knowing I was breaking the medical code of 'as prescribed', leaving me short on the last leg of my unrefillable prescription. At the end of my rope, I was left with the only viable option for relief; to visit the ever-friendly and accessible liquor store, where I would find my drink or choice, the obscure cordial Cream Sherry that would soothe my nerves for a few hours until the poison of the excessively sweet potion I could drink uncontrollably like water would poison my body: headaches, nausea, paralyzing anxiety/depression due to lack of ability to obtain proper sleep (restless hours wrestling with unmade day time bedding) and the inability to eat.

My normally conservative consumption or American Spirits "organic" elite cigarettes would increase from a conservatively regulated 3 fags a day to 7 - 10, as if the process of procuring a fresh cigarette from a pack, lighting it, drawing the first wave of smoke into my lungs, feel the nicotine course through my body, retiring to my designated 'smoking lounge' chair with a clean ashtray like I was a guest on a 1970's smoke-friendly televised talk show, and engage the homeopathic air purifier to neutralize the smoke pollution was one of my only logically cognitive solutions to my uncontrollably restless anxiety.

I would crush and snort Xanax pills before attending an AA meeting, convening with other sober cigarette smokers in the parking lot of a scheduled meeting, and actively participating in the practices at these congergations, interacting with seemingly happy sober colleagues for an hour, bookended with small talk and another cigarette in the parking lot before would I return home to snort another crushed Xanax pill. It was my way, the highway, which I did not lose any sleep over. Just another deception I had mastered and did not feel hangdog about. I would inevitably run out of my Xanax half-way through the monthly prescription, which my gluttonous addict mind never seemed to master. Jonesing from benzos was paralyzingly painful. Dr. RxXnX started acting suspicious when I asked for an increase in dose. I never revealed my complete substance abuse history to this general practitioner who was treating the medical disorder I came to him looking for relief from as a growing anxiety, and he provided the medicine. I told him I heroically had chosen to abstain from alcohol consumption, which I never alluded to there ever having been a problem in the consumption of, enlightening the Doctor that I wanted to give the Xanax an unadulterated chance to work on my anxiety. Dr. RxXnX would never have prescribed Xanax to me if he knew of my documented substance abuse and institutionalizations. But once I was given Xanax, and I consumed more than prescribed daily, my body developed a physiological addiction to the narcotic benzos in Xanax that when depleted and the next appointment to refill was one – two weeks away, the jonesing my mind, body, and spirit experienced was paralyzing.

Benzodiazepines are a type of medication known as tranquilizers: Ativan, Valium, Klonopin, and Xanax. While they are some of the most commonly prescribed medications in the United States, most patients do not have the addictive disposition to abuse them, able to maintain a vial in their medicine chest for months with no need to refill as they only take when needed, if ever. But given my predilection for mind altering substances, I can take more than prescribed playing dumb to the price I would pay when there are no more. My Doctor prescribed monthly supply of Xanax was turning into drug abuse. I couldn't eat, sleep, or socialize. I could barely get the nerve to make my one short daily phone check-in with my BF, unable to articulate how uncomfortable I felt. The suffering. The guilt of gluttony of consuming my prescription, leaving no alternative than to suffer through the detox alone, or, buy my drink of choice, a liter of Cream Sherry, to alleviate the discomfort and depression at least for a few hours.

After 11 years of living in the posh studio in the exclusive high-rise apartment building I was blessed to call a home during my residence in the city of Poughkeepsie, I realized it was time to move from the fascist colony where I never broke a rule, but was the subject of a lot of gossip about my illicit lifestyle, all of it speculation with not an ounce of truth. In 2013, I had written a memoir about my glamorous life of arriving in sex-saturated Times Square in 1976 at the innocent age of 18 years old, on the very day I was driven by my estranged parents to the college of my choice, Stony Brook University, where I deposited my footlocker of clothes in my new dorm only to excuse myself from Freshman orientation to take the Long Island Railroad into Penn Station and hike to the vortex of sexual hedonism beckoning me from the flashing lights of 42nd Street movie theaters up to the historic row of bars and restaurant known as Tin Pan Alley. Blessed or cursed, I was picked up by a young humpy male hustler not much older than me in years but wiser in life experiences, introduced to my first man-on-man sexual activity, and summarily convinced by new gay mentor to successfully audition and commit to working as a male stripper at the most respectable and well-run gay establishment in the otherwise shady adult entertainment businesses of Times Square; the Gaiety Male Burlesque Theater. That moment is vivid and vital to my coming out as a homosexual as most heterosexual males' virgin sexual intercourse with a woman. I was encouraged by friends to write my story, which evolved from Times Square and Stony Brook University to a successful social and occupational life experiencing some of the best underground and renown discotheques in NYC from 1976 – 2004, when I crashed and burned from the excess of my substance fueled narcissistic lifestyle. I wrote my first book in two months, submitted my carefully enticing introductory "Query" synopsis of *Homo GoGo Man: A Fairytale About A Boy Who Grew Up In Discoland* to 50 publishing agencies I selected as appropriate for the book's LGBT subject matter, and astonishingly offered a standard publishing contract with DonnaInk Publishing within one month. Blessed. I was able to take a pipe-dream of becoming a published writer to reality in three months, when the impression I got was that people get stuck, distracted, and disillusioned from completing their first novel, their first painting, their first offspring after years of false starts, languishing in their disappointment as untalented, unobtainable, barren, dashing their dream creating something of interest to the general public. Artist require a strong backbone. But a published book available in big-box book stores and the world wide web does not sell without the author promoting the book, or more specifically the blogging about first-hand experience of the historic details as a survivor of the well-documented era of hedonistic NYC before it was white-washed for tourism and family consumption during the late 1990's. So, I began blogging about all the storied clubs, the evolution of popular mind-altering drugs, the explosive social and legal success of the once rag tag gay revolution, and of course the ever-popular celebrity gossip. My publisher had never considered the now burgeoning clout of gay consumerism, so my book was a first risk she took to represent material categorized as LGBT. I classified my book as a memoir, a personal cautionary tale about the dangers of narcissism and addictive hedonism in pre-gentrified NYC. My Orlando, Florida publishing company's conservative home-base gamble on publishing my book paid off, years before the horrific mass slaughter of innocent human beings by a deranged sexually confused gun toting maniac in the very same otherwise Disney World devoted locale of central Florida. Four and a half years later, the book is still a success, to her publishing company and to my fans around the world. It was my pride and joy to finally classify myself as an author; as close to being an artist as I could only have dreamed of when I was excelling in art class in elementary school.

But I knew that I needed to be in NYC to personal promote my book, not for profit, but for exposure. I had outgrown the limitations of culturally empty Poughkeepsie, got tired of my ever-greedy landlord's yearly attempt to financially rape me with above market rental leases with no fringe benefits.

My kitchen was equipped with the very same appliances installed when the luxury apartment high-rise was built in 1972, coated in the then popular gold, which 40 years later were still working, but ready to die at any given moment. I came to my senses that my tremendous credit card debt was due to my devotion to restore my 1969 Nova muscle car, so I sold it to wash out the debt, preparing me to exit the Hudson Valley to live in civil commitment with my BF of 6 solid years, Storm Orion, in his long-term residence in the outskirts of a borough of NYC I never familiarized myself with, Jamaica, Queens, New York City.

I milked the opportunity to make one last long drive in a rental car to Mount Kisco to obtain one last vial of Xanax as prescribed by Dr. RxXnX, not revealing that this would be our final visit before moving to Queens. I had already begun my 'google' search for "New York City Doctor Prescription Xanax Anxiety" to satisfy my physiological as well as psychological addiction to the narcotic of benzodiazepines. I had left NYC in 2004, believing that the city would be a blight to my chance to quietly live out my golden years in sober tranquility, and here I was, returning to the city that I believed I had burnt all bridges with my unemployability, lack of financial resources, dissolving friendships, and an unrecognizable new skyline that became the hungry obsession of luxury apartment building developers out-shadowing the brunt of tasteless monopoly held by an entitled Queens boy who won the fortuitous lottery of success, President Donald J. Trump. It was no longer the city that never sleeps; it was now the city that no one could afford to live in.

CHAPTER 10
Acute Xanax Abuse

I met my current reigning life partner at Riis Beach in the Rockaways, Brooklyn, New York, one Sunday summer afternoon in 1999. He had the tenacity and assertiveness to approach my otherwise snobbish public presence to make my acquaintance, which impressed and flattered me, given how strikingly handsome, albeit inappropriate our age disparity. His sexual barometer was peaking at the youthful age of 27 while I had crossed into a very well-preserved middle age of 41; a 14-year age difference that transfers to practically an entire generation gap. He passed my discriminatory cross-examination as a suitable carnal partner, with not much left to my sexual imagination given that the only garment this dark-skinned Adonis modeled was a small red swimsuit. I was willing to give him my phone number to schedule a future playdate, with the caveat that I was already in a relationship with another man but was unhappily unappreciated by this absent active drug addict. Ergo, my solitary presence at the beach after yet another weekend feeling like a widow as my drug addled boyfriend was Missing in Action. I would be damned to sit by the phone waiting for his call or rebuff the advances of a flattering stranger. So, if my picture-perfect suitor in a red speedo was willing to accept these circumstances, I would entertain an affair with this young, dark and lovely boy-toy with the exotic name "Storm Orion".

Storm was a seriously talented singer and song writer, professionally train-ed by a vocal coach, represented by an agent, and had a recorded his own songs as well as performed backup for more successful artists. He was vigor-ously determined to successfully succeed in the volatile music industry. After attending one of his live performances at a reputable downtown venue, 'Joe's Pub', on Lafayette Street, where Storm appeared onstage barefoot, shirtless, clad in nothing but a pair of tight brown leather pants that matched his Panamanian complexion accompanied by a trio of formally dressed instru-mentalists, that I fell from sexually attracted to full tilt love for this man. When a person can express himself effectively with an innate talent, it can ignite a hotspot in the brain of the spectator, comparable to the euphoria activated by a psychoactive drug of choice.

As the spectacle of my dead-end relationship with my legitimate boy-friend and the third wheel, Crystal Meth, got more dangerously melo-dramatic, I had to give naïve Storm his walking papers to spare him from what I was afraid was going to get ugly. Verbal and physically violent alterca-tions erupted, involving police intervention, an anesthetized increase in my own substance abuse, unemployability and financial bankruptcy inciting my ridiculous plan of escaping from all my problems, especially my sadomaso-chistic relationship, by selling off all my valuable material possessions after 25 years of living and excelling in New York City to escape to Greece, expecting to start a new life, relying on the upcoming 2004 Summer Olym-pics to be hosted in Athens. I spent two nights in terribly overpriced hotels in Athens losing my gumption to seek employment in the upcoming interna-tional sporting event because my American ethnocentricity had not consid-ered that my lack of communicating in the native language of the city where the Olympics originated (776 BC) would be such an obstacle that I bailed on that pipe dream. I escaped Athens to where I had earlier pleasurable experiences and knew I could integrate with English speaking visitors on the once jetsetter now gay magnet of the Greek island of Mykonos. I spent 3 months hotel-hopping on this self-indulgent destination with nothing but my corporate American Express card that was in payment default, but bull-shitted my way through credit extensions to pay my hotel bills and in-house meals, dancing away the reality that all foolish ideas eventually lead to a rude awakening . I was rudely made aware that the summer, and therefore the tourist industry of Mykonos, was at a close as I awoke from my hotel room to the disruptive noise of laborers vigorously removing outdoor patio furniture scheduled for storage. I made a hasty departure from the summer island of escapism embarrassingly devoid of any other straggling visitors but myself, and lied to American Express customer service to approve the cost of my return airfare under the guise that my "partner" was suddenly hospitalized with Acquired Immune Deficiency Syndrome, and perpetuated my financial scam that I needed to abruptly end what I falsely qualified as an international business trip (it was a "corporate card" issued to a business I had created and legally incorporated; an unprofitable production company in film location-friendly Williamsburg, Brooklyn). It amazes me how low my substance abuse is willing to allow me to maneuver my otherwise respectable code of conduct.

Back in NYC, with no place to call my home, I turned to the very reason I escaped to Greece; my co-dependency to my drug-addled boyfriend, Sharif, who gladly took me into his home, relishing his success at reacquiring my masochistic devotion to him. He was on his own diminishing financial, physical, and mental health fall from his once noble respectability from the fickle society of NYC gays. He was the source of malicious and mostly true gossip. His charlatan act worked, and then it didn't. Drugs, even that which seemed to empower the user enough to rank as their drug of choice, have their run until the substance doesn't work anymore, and the devil seeks his restitution. Sharif died after a failed attempt to kill himself consuming toxic household cleaning products, bailed out of the suicide by calling for help himself, recovered in Saint Vincent's hospital with enough positive TLC to believe he could continue his blessed life clean and sober, only to make one final deadly pact with the devil by partaking in not his nemesis drug of choice Crystal Meth, but a substitute that would make his conscious believe he was not breaking his long fought for sober survival; he overdosed on Ketamine (Special K), placing his euphoric seeking body and mind into a coma that left his person too weak to recover from, and was pronounced dead after 8 days. I was busy running from my own death demon by demeaning my once independent and financially solvent character by couch surfing amongst my weary friends as I returned to the one means of income that I knew did not require me to abstain from alcohol or drug consumption while performing my job: I was a go-go man at the age of 46. I was stubbornly resistant to attend Sharif's memorial service, much less visit his coma-induced body in the hospital as I received updates from one of his friends who acknowledged the once intimate and long-term relationship I had with this dying man. I never had closure, which I am punished for to this day with nightmare's consisting of hopelessly ceaseless dramatic emotional and physical scenarios with my long dead ex-lover, Sharif. I wake up in a disoriented panic. Post-Traumatic Stress Syndrome. It was understandable that I was destined to follow my tragic ex-lover's footsteps with my own dangerous dance with drug death, and that prophecy came to fruition only 6 months later, in January 2004.

However, I was spared. A cruel joke or an earnest symbol of his ever-sincere love for me, Sharif is one of my celestial guardian angels who I privately communicate with, in good times and bad. This was the ugly situation I was savvy enough to spare Storm Orion any involvement much less witness to.

I lived my renewed life in respite from NYC after recovering from my self-induced devastation in 2004. As rich as my new life was considering how low I had allowed my substance abuse to take me, I could never find a sexual partner to satisfy my elitist standards in upstate New York, 70 miles from the gay mecca of New York City. I flirted with "straight" men who found me entertaining, even titillating, but I was smart enough to realize that the hunt is more satisfying than the actual conquest. So, I was sexually celibate for 8 semi-sober years before I thought I would reach out to the wild card I kept in my hope chest. I did some internet research to locate and reach out to Storm Orion, my sexual boy-toy, eleven years after imposing a separation. I was willing to grant that his fine self was already spoken for, and I would be summarily rejected. But to my good fortune, and the serendipity of life, he was single, alone, and insisted that he was waiting for my overdue call. It turns out that as much as both of our glamorous self-indulgent lives had been through the lowest pits of despair, we were both repaired damaged goods, perfectly matched to secure an honest adult relationship based on unconditional support and a little cheerleading to not give up on our dreams that both of us one time "it" boys were now realistically willing to leave behind as fond memories in our pasts and live humbly in domestic bliss together. Love on a daily basis, without the pressure of extracting an erection, can be gently gratifying with a partner to weather the reality of mortality.

Storm and I maintained a long-distance relationship with monthly conjugal visits every month as I lived in Poughkeepsie and he in Jamaica Queens, and subsisted on daily phone calls that contained a dose of life-affirming human interaction from a caring listener as well as the unpredictably powerful momentum of unexpected phone sex. We were ready to cohabitate daily, and I was ready to return to my hometown of NYC. I had performed what in recovery is labeled a "geographical" to set a new fresh course in my life. I would leave the Hudson Valley and move back to NYC, under the justifycation that it would be better to promote my book. Given his large apartment combined with my acquired taste for clean modern home aesthetics, and we able to make a comfortable, eye-pleasing home that satisfied my concession to always expect more out of life. My family adores Storm, not just for his sweet honest charm that is appreciated as sincerity in my family of high expectations, but for the balance he apparently provides to my otherwise tumultuous personality. Both equally handsome and artistically talented, we are opposites in demeanor, which I believe is the secret to our success as a conflict-free committed couple. He is the Yin to my Yang.

When I got to NYC, I found a doctor on the internet who seemed like a perfect fit for the medical relationship I needed; a renewal of the prescription for Xanax I last legally filled with Dr. RxXnx in now unreachable Mount Kisco. My new drug of choice provider was located under a 'Google' search of keywords: 'legal prescription Xanax doctor NYC'. There was no investigation or questions regarding past substance abuse history. For the exorbitant price of $200. for a 10 minute visit with the doctor, I sat in a small waiting room with standing room only with what looked like well-groomed and accessorized 20-something millenniums fixated on their smart phones, all looking uncomfortable and exhibiting obvious anti-social body language as we jockeyed for the limited seating in the shabby waiting room for an hour or more to get our fix. I thought we should interact, support each other, but the ambience was one of humiliating withdrawal that we were all there, under not so respectable circumstances. It was like waiting to score with a drug dealer, only with a long queue ahead of you. It was a drug mill. It was far from legitimately professional. It was an illicit medical practice. But I got my

Xanax script which thankfully was not ever questioned or rejected by the financially motivated doctor or the pharmacist.

But the dose as prescribed was never enough for me, and I would run out in less than two weeks. So, I found another Doctor online willing to treat me for anxiety, this one in a more reputable office / institution (NYU Langone) and offered as a more pleasant and professional visit. I was charged the bargain price of only $100 a visit due to my financial/insurance situation that qualified my out of pocket cost for the visit on the gracious NYC / Langone sliding scale. So, I had two NYC doctors that I would see in one month to double my dose. This worked out for a few months until I was humiliated to be confronted by the more respectable doctor at NYU / Langone who left me chagrined when he confronted me with evidence of his knowledge that I was double dating doctors. Instead of ending our professional relationship, he was willing to solve the equation by increasing my monthly dose under the promise I would not return to the drug mill doctor's office. It was a win-win situation. Except I still could not exercise discipline with my daily dose of Xanax. I would run out, freak out, drink, and got resourceful and dangerous by searching for black market Xanax on Craigslist, a practice I read and stored in my memory from an article about this currently popular activity amongst the citizens of this sophisticated metropolis in 'New York' Magazine.

In 1976, my introduction to recreational drugs by street savvy co-workers at the Gaiety included an introduction to a face and a residence to obtain mind-altering substances that felt safe from the law, and a pleasant interaction with another gay disco bunny. Once I was vetted by these recreational dealers who could evaluate my character as a respectable and financially reliable customer, I was given direct access to the dealer's home phone number to make appointments to visit when I needed to stock up on whatever was the drug of choice in the dance clubs we all frequented. Cash, no credit. And no outrageous behavior as this was the home of a hard-working professional who augmented his income by selling drugs to safe contacts on the side. It was like he was an Avon salesperson in his free time. I was never without a drug contact and prided myself in never having to take a chance buying questionable substances on the dangerous streets, much less in a crowded discotheque. Besides, I liked having drugs in my possession before going to a club, sparing the anxious search for leads on who had what in a dark and mysterious club. I was once an entitled drug user.

Now back in NYC in 2016, the city and the protocol of obtaining drugs was very different. Sometimes my source for Xanax initiated by a listing in Craigslist would be with street drug thugs under potentially criminally dangerous circumstances to feed my daily benzo addiction, and I was aware that what I was buying and ingesting from these unreliable sources was probably not always the real McCoy, but a bootleg version or worse a bogus facsimile of the medication; worthless paste. I would be forced to sweat it out, abstaining from alcohol knowing the poisonous reaction my body, mind and soul would produce the day after consuming a liter of cream sherry, leaving me more debilitated and hopeless waiting for a text from my street dealers that Xanax was once again available. It wasn't like I had a renewal prescription. These instances of deep hopelessness would not even inspire me to make the effort to answer the ringing phone much less travel to the dealer's residence of substance. I was paralyzed, acutely depressed, and demonstrated this pathetically to my dear supportive and too understanding boyfriend who I shared a home and my sometimes-pathetic life with.

During the first winter upon returning to NYC to promote my book and cohabitate with my perfect boyfriend, I suffered through a long drought of street 'Xanax', struggling with acute benzodiazepine withdrawal, unable to eat or sleep, paralyzed in our apartment located along a noisy thoroughfare in Jamaica, Queens, anxious from the persistent noise pollution of alarms from firetrucks, ambulances and police patrol cars rushing to another human being's crisis. I thought I was going to go insane, climaxing into a second nightmare of deciding the only solution was to end my life. My boyfriend, Storm, who was blessed with a zero tolerance for mind-altering substances, was sleeping peacefully in the bedroom that I could not find sleep much less peace with. My mind went mad, resigned to the fact that suicide was my only salvation. I had read about a rash of hangings performed successfully by celebrity designers: Alexander McQueen, Kate Spade, and L'Wren Scott (better known as Mike Jagger's girlfriend than her fashion business). So I took a foot stool, a strong leather belt, and dashed out of our apartment to the stairwell, only to be face a disgusting molding wall that appeared to be streaming a waterfall of toxic liquid, which was revolting enough to eliminate this location that had all the correct architectural structures to perform a hanging, only the ambience was off. If that was not enough to nix the hanging in my boyfriend's apartment building, unbeknownst to me I stepped into the jurisdiction of a motion detector, intended to keep transient visitors from congregating in the hallways, sending an ear piercing alarm that sent me scrambling out of the stairwell in horror with my hanging paraphernalia to return to the ironic sanctity of my boyfriend's apartment.

Restless and frustrated, conscious of the deadly hour of 4:00 AM with no chance of a pardon to survive the night alive, I did what I my historical instincts told me to do; grab a butcher knife from the kitchen and lay in the dry bathtub, tracing patterns on my already scarred arms, now decoratively tattooed with unique tribal designs that I referred to as 'cuffs', leaving a white line of a scratch on the surface of my forearms without breaking the skin.

I suppose I was tired of playing the suicide charade by myself, and eventually woke my peacefully sleeping BF Storm to expose myself not as his better half but as a suicidal maniac that was directionless and needed an audience to perform my hysteria. At one point, I was playing a cat and mouse game with him, now that I had an audience, by making manic attempts to open one of our sixth floor windows threatening to jump, find more butcher knifes, box cutters, anything sharp, lock myself in the bathroom, all under the quiet radar of not disturbing or involving our building neighbors. After a one hour performance, I was physically too exhausted to play hide and go kill myself with my sweet boyfriend thwarting me, and let the voice of reason convince me that I needed to go the hospital, specifically the Emergency Room, as I was having a "panic" attack. I could not articulate a complete sentence, and my whole body jolted every few seconds from muscle spasms.

It was 5:00am on that all too familiar late Saturday night debacle, advancing into an early Sunday morning that I sought the hope of relief from my mental disorder due to acute benzo withdrawal which provoked my otherwise cognitively well-tuned mind to entertain notions of suicide, revisiting a nightmarish night I was a veteran of 15 years earlier, and documented in detail at the beginning of this tragic story with good intentions. Like addiction, the possibility of relapse is ever more probable with each recurrence of the event.

My emotionally grounded boyfriend allowed me to dissolve into a nebulous entity, unable to articulate what I wanted or needed, much less make the commitment to seek professional medical help. But his pious and persistently patient presence invoked the motivation for me to agree that I needed to get out of the apartment that was already a tainted prison of restlessness, and after a five minute cab ride with my mind selfishly projecting that my suffering was the only pain felt on all of the planet Earth, we arrived at the Emergency Room intake desk where two seemingly calm, cool, and collected staff personnel allowed me to stutter and stammer my reason for being there. I know that I mentioned "acute Xanax withdrawal" and "multiple attempts at suicide" and "paralyzing heart palpitations", but I never felt such loss of control of my auditory skills, not to mention the uncontrollable twerks and twitches my otherwise graceful and socially conscious body was exhibiting. I felt like Linda Blair, possessed by a demon presence, in "the Exorcist". Storm stood by, my Rock of Gibraltar, following up my melodramatic introductory performance with the administrative information required by the hospital: name, address, age, emergency contact, relevant medical history, and medical insurance status. I was instructed to take a seat in a civil manner, where I continue to restlessly wrestle with what I had convinced myself were uninvited demons possessing me to make a public spectacle, so unlike the self-conscious entitled mask and costume I was accustomed to fooling the general public into believing was my envious and invincible self, I was no longer a proud figurine atop a Prom King trophy.

Within 10 interminable minutes, my name was called to partake in the important first stage of the life-saving purpose of the Emergency Room. An obviously tired and professionally unchallenged intake nurse responsible for obtaining each new ER patients vital human body statistics to classify their threat to mortality reprimanded me to stop what I could not or would not seem to control; my herky-jerky body spasms that were preventing her from efficiently performing her job. I promised to behave, internally scolding myself for not having better self-control, and let the entry-level voice of authority of a tired, overworked, unsympathetic intake nurse scores a victory over my choice to lose control.

I was then instructed to "rest" on a gurney in a small hallway that connected the ER entrance for patients arriving from EMS vehicles that had the license to ignore all of the rules of the road meant ensure vehicular safety to be swept passed the hospital hospitality desk and intake nurse I had already invested what I thought was precious time to be relieved of my biblically proportioned suffering. The small hallway I was awkwardly and mysteriously instructed to "rest" in (impossibly incongruous to my state of restlessness) was also the site of the security desk, manned by two uniformed and armed New York City Police officers, prepared for any possible threat of violence erupting in the ER, apparent in their cagy and suspicious attention to me and any non-hospital staff that was in their immediate vicinity.

It wasn't long before I could process and project what was beginning to feel like was a carnival house ride through unexpected rooms of new surprises strapped to my gurney as I was wheeled through the next set of doors to the architecturally single silo that was the Emergency Room. It gave me the impression of images both real and theatrically created to portray the Mission Control center for a space launch enterprise, like NASA. Circular in design, concentric circles of monitors, processors, containers and file cabinets being opened and closed and restocked at the pace of a fast food franchise, and a daisy chain of patients positioned along the outer extremes of the circumference of the room.

An intravenous injection with a feeding tube was administered to my inner arm at the bend of the elbow to provide what I wished would be a sedative but was only an innocuous clear substance (concentrated and supplemented water) to hydrate what the hospital assumed was a dehydrated body after prolonged drug and/or alcohol consumption. I drink water like a rain forest, motivated by the theory that a healthy adult human body should maintain 60 percent water, which upon depletion leads to the unattractive side effects of aging: wrinkles, greying hair, and low muscle index.

I was summarily approached by male ER attendant of no apparent medical authority other than to be assigned my ER guardian, who inhumanely instructed me to undress from my street clothes that were packed into a large brown disposable bag reminiscent of a heavy duty sack to fill with raked leaves after autumn's funeral service when trees can no longer could sustain their life, to be orphaned and left dead and unwanted on the ground below. Granted possession of only my own personal underpants, in my case a pair of boxers less publicly humiliating than white briefs, I was presented with a disposable paper-like shapeless hospital smock, barely covering my torso, with no sleeves, as short as a miniskirt, and worn backwards, with the opening exposing my back. Once again relegated to my assigned gurney, chained by the IV tube in my arm attached to the elevated hydration fluid sack, I was positioned along the wall of the ER room like during the land prospecting pioneer Americans of the 18th century venturing westward would position their horse drawn wagons to encircle the family encampments as the first line of defense for protection from unpredictable threats.

I noticed there was a segregation in the population of patients in the ER based on the color of the hospital gown assigned to wear by the ER staff. Those in need of priority medical attention were wearing red. Those of us seeking mental attention (mental disorder, substance abuse overdose, suicide attempts) were basically made to feel like we were taking up space in the life-saving ER, being "observed" from our relegated gurney, and were assigned to wear purple hospital gowns. The significance of distinct wardrobe color assignments was not lost on me, familiar with the book, movie, and cable TV series "The Handmaid's Tale". In this futuristic apocalyptic tale, the 'Handmaids', sexually enslaved outcasts of society, are required to wear red dresses, while the barren wives of the male-dominated ruling class wear blue.

Purple, the color I had been taught was associated with "mental madness", as well as the 'color of choice' for royalty, distinguished those patients in the ER that were being monitored for psyche evaluation. With no literature to read (I was not in possession of my reading glasses) and no televisions that would interfere with the multitude of screens monitoring vital signs as well as patient inventory spreadsheets indicating bed number, assigned doctor, and updated vital statistics that I watched like a traveler at an airport waiting for my respective scheduled flight update, I lost track of how long I was left unattended in the ER, making me very restless not knowing when some attention and action was going to be paid to me, with very little there was to do to pass the time. It seemed like 12 hours since I was instructed to remain on my gurney until I was finally introduced to the obviously case-overloaded hospital psyche ward liaison who cheerfully explained that I would be moved from the pointlessness of remaining in a state of perpetual ignorance by the ER staff to the more appropriate psyche ward environment and respective staff. When he asked how I was doing, I

frankly told the liaison that I was very restless and anxious for some medicinal relief, i.e.: a sedative of some kind that surely the hospital was well
equipped with. I was promised an Ativan, a mild variation of Xanax, which
I took as an oral contract by this sole authority of my circumstances in this
otherwise alienating medical ER. Just like in a crowded club looking for my
knight in shining armor to sweep me off my feet to the seduction of his
castle, I kept a hawk-eye for this otherwise benign looking man, expecting
him to return with a sedative as promised, only to have my hopes dashed as
he never returned for what seemed like an agonizing couple of hours, nes
pas the promised Ativan. I emotionally, physiologically, and psychologically
Jonesing.

I was conscious of more patients admitted to the ER, some in the company of civilian police officers, to be stripped of their street clothes and
marked as "crazy" when presented with a purple hospital gown. Many of
these newly arriving compatriots made their mad presence known by arguing
with the hospital staff and required some physical restraint from the lingering
police officers. As frustrated, impatient, and judgmental as I was about the
futility of my extended and wasted hours limited to remaining on my gurney,
I was polite and respectful of any infinitesimal interaction granted by any ER
staff, believing that maybe this sobering nightmare might be dismissed with
my trustworthy experience of charm.

It was a full 14 hours since I had convinced my caring boyfriend who was
out of his league to handle my desperate hissy fit to accompany me to the
ER when he deserved to getting a peaceful night's sleep before the psyche
liaison returned to my captive presence without the promised seductively
sedative medicine, to instruct me to follow him through a series of familiar
entranceways monitored by a wall phone to open, close, and re-lock like a
series of canals to reach the wing of the hospital accommodating the psyche
ward, seemingly far removed from the medical facility, like a leper colony.
When we reached what was furnished as a waiting room, I was instructed to
sit, which I performed with as much dignity and masculinity to mask my
modesty of wearing only my public appropriate boxers and my purple hospital gown barely covering my otherwise naked body, which I struggled with
pulling down to cover my legs like a woman wearing a street appropriate
short dress that naturally hikes up when seated, like on a television talk show.

I was also trembling from the cold winter weather, inappropriately dressed for the winter season even though I was indoors. When my person was transferred by paperwork from the liaison to a beefy bodyguard intake officer employed by the psyche ward, I was given my first display of compassion when my new bodyguard took one look at me and barked to the liaison that I should not have been brought to his guardianship in the humiliating and temperature inappropriate hospital gown, and that I should have been offered more modest coverage, and that my personal street clothes I wore when admitted to ER should be in my possession, now that I am a resident of the psyche ward. The beefy bodyguard apologized for the debacle as if I was a person who deserved some dignity. He quickly summoned for proper hospital attire (a pajama set, booties, and a robe) before presenting me to the resident psychologist for an extensive diagnostic intake. By now, my 14-year history of psych treatment, and my gift for articulating myself thoroughly with long, self-deprecating, sometimes tangential declamations, made me a long-winded talker. I had nothing to hide.

That was the last I saw of a highly educated authority on mental health with impressive credentials during my emergency trip to the hospital, just like when I was last transferred from a hospital ER for an attempted/threat of suicide in 2004. I was then released like a rescue animal into the unorganized and seemingly unsupervised confines of the Jamaica Hospital Psyche ward. Unlike my prior deployment, this psyche ward was a self-contained single-story structure, eliminating any reference to the "Flight Deck". But the ambience was the same. No windows to see the world outside, no structured activities, and no personal itinerary for a patient to ask and receive help. The psyche ward was manned by a seemingly bored and unsocial supervisory staff (I must have visited the bathroom a multitude of times without their consent or knowledge to examine the blemish prone face I had been obsessed with examining in my apartment bathroom mirror for the past 5 days), where, left to my own devices, could have perhaps harmed myself.

Just like the detox in Poughkeepsie, I realized that the Queens Hospital psyche ward served no other purpose than to contain the patient in a lockdown ward with no structure to pass the time other than to sleep, something that seemed to come naturally to what appeared to be unfocused humans who found sleep easily and preferred it to interacting with other patients or staff. I was still too focused, obsessed being an active participant in the game of life. The staff in the psyche ward clearly hated their jobs. They only talked to each other, complaining about this or that employment condition, and their lack of verbal interaction with the patients led me to believe that they weren't even trained on how to perform their job effectively. It was an entry level medical work-study program for the staff of the psyche ward. No books or TV were provided to distract the detainees from literally climbing the windowless walls. I did not want to interact with any of the other patients, although I will always remember the young gregarious woman who manipulated the ER staff to allow her to remain in her street attire, use the hospital phone to make numerous personal calls, leading me to believe she was a journalist. The next time I saw her she was in the same hospital pajama set that I was modeling as she cheerfully socialized with whoever would have the patience to deal with her apparent high-maintenance personality in the psyche ward. The black man brought in handcuffs by police officers to the ER who went ballistic when he realized that his fate was now being reduced to a stay in the psyche ward protested by stripping himself nude to the shock of the hospital staff as well as us conscious residents in the ER, until he was forced into a locked room for solitary confinement. I encountered his subdued, sedated presence in the psyche ward. They were noteworthy players in the undesirable theater that I swore I would never return to, but being the protagonist of my own storyline, here I was again, institutionalized, for the third time in 15 years of my so-called entitled life. I had only myself to blame for my circumstances, and no one but myself to advocate to expedite my return to my well-deserved life of free will in the land of liberty and the pursuit of happiness.

The staff was not worth approaching about any other matter than the monotony of structured mealtimes, especially given the fact that it was the weekend, where the more senior and preferred staff were enjoying their well-deserved time off duty, leaving little if no professionally qualified psyche personnel for me to seek out for a serious conversation about my individual circumstances and my intention to advocate for my quick approval to be discharged after 24 hours of observation. Witnessing my desperate decision to have my BF Storm leave the comfort of our home to accompany me to the ER 28 hours earlier was another lesson that I did not want to be reminded of as one of the many clichés recited in AA: the definition of insanity is repeating the same behavior while expecting different results. In my case, I was cognizant that the consequences of my actions were getting worse.

I needed to initiate some intelligent connections with the ruling staff to acquire a fair hearing that I was knowledgeable would be effective in my not being lost in the land of the unfocused and advocate for my earliest convenient discharge based on the strong case I knew would be convincing and was based on truth, so it would be all the more persuasive.

As I sat in the psyche ward's cafeteria aware of the presence of the young African American man who offered a shocking but effective demonstration of his frustration and anger regarding his incarcerated circumstances upon admission to the ER, handcuffed and guarded by two uniformed police officers, by stripping bare naked was now exhibiting a deep state of major depression, sobbing uncontrollably as a local TV news program peppered their broadcast with the usual "blood and guts" stories that may not be more important than what is happening in Washington, DC, much less the World, but keeps the sensation-seeking audience's attention. The overly emotional response of the young man compared with his aggressive behavior in ER indicated that he might be bi-polar to exhibit such extreme mood swings. Nobody, even the high-spirited female facsimile of a journalist cum psyche ward patient that I also observed for lack of anything else to do felt warranted or humane enough to offer her moral support to a colleague obviously exhibiting a mental breakdown beyond any of the psyche ward staff's limited ability. An on-resident MSW hospital staff member was dispatched to perform his graduate school training and innate listening skills to pacify the emotionally troubled patient. I saw my ticket out of the indeterminate sentence of the futility of the psyche ward by making a connection with the visiting MSW. I waited until he had used his soft voice and calming mantras to stabilize my troubled psyche colleague. I politely reached out to the MSW to ask if he had a few minutes to allow me to communicate my circumstances and convince him of my inevitable privilege to be discharged ASAP based on my convincing credentials: I was already enrolled and attending an outpatient substance abuse program at the LGBT Center in the West Village, I lived with and was accompanied to and would be the guardian receiving me upon discharge from the psyche ward, and that I had no medical insurance to pay for the exorbitant cost of spending another day in the hospital. Serendipity, the MSW, who was performing rare weekend duty at the hospital, was not only listening to me without judgement, heard my sincerity and knowledge on the circumstances, and when I provided my BFs name and contact information, proved what a small world it is when the MSW expressed excitement that he knew Storm professionally and personally, and not only was an admirer of his fine nature, but the fact that I was cohabitating with this upstanding citizen was the final testimony that I would be better at home than to spend another hour, much less a day, in the futility of the psyche ward. I was never so happy to see Storm waiting for me at the intake / discharge waiting room, like I was being pardoned from execution and released from prison. Storm was bestowed my custody by the MSW who now knew us both personally like a marital judge joining the hands of a newly wedded couple till death do them part. I was also informed by the MSW that the hospital neighboring our Jamaica home provided an outpatient substance abuse program that might be a good, if nothing other than convenient, new commitment to my otherwise exhausted outpatient attendance at the LGBT Center, which I had reached the predictable 6 month gestation period of enthusiastically participated in, emotionally resenting and resisting, both staff and fellow clients.

Once I graciously retired from my association with the LGBT Center Outpatient program and became a regular client at the Queens hospital outpatient program, I became aware of the myriad of services, clinical (mental) as well as medical (physical) that I needed to start addressing, utilizing all of the available services on my uninsured bargain priced sliding scale. Blessed and Charmed.

After explaining my story to my outpatient case manager, it was suggested that I revisit attention to my physical wellbeing as I had not been examined by a medical doctor in decades, and I was approaching my 60th birthday. Initially concerned about the damage from long term drug and alcohol abuse would reveal itself in blood work. I put on a good front like on all my important interviews to impress the doctor with dazzling exterior (good genes, hygiene, diet, fit muscularly developed physique, proper hygiene, and well dressed), but the blood work results would reveal excessively high levels of cholesterol, which was an indication of my disposition to cardiovascular failure. My father suffered his first of many heart attacks at age 70, requiring open heart surgery, a Defibrillator implant that expired after reaching its quota of providing life-saving countershocks (like a dead battery), and after 10 years of too many doctors' opinions and ER visits, and "do not resuscitate" orders, advocated to no longer waste his precious time and money on the quagmire of the medical community and convalesce at his home with his wife and family and a weekly visit from a hospice worker, who he resented the presence of. I am my father's son. I am now able to provide my health care providers with family history that is more telling than any blood work. But the high cholesterol level did open the door for me to be referred to the Cardiology department to be tested for any indication of irregular heart condition through a series of four separate heart tests.

Of the 4 heart exams, wearing a Holter heart monitor ankle bracelet for 24 hours provided the definitive proof that my heart had two separate instances of irregularity. This was enough evidence for the cardiologist to classify me at high risk for cardiovascular failure, with medication to address my condition, and the reassuring advice that if I should ever find myself feeling like I am suffering from intense heart palpitations, that any visit to an ER should NOT be classified as a stigmatizing "panic attack", but as "heart attack", to receive proper and professional treatment for a potentially life-threatening condition. I'm not just a "nut" case. I am predisposed to cardiovascular failure like my father suffered, fought, and eventually succumbed to. I was prescribed a moderate daily dose of a beta-blocker designed to decrease the effect of adrenaline to the heart, cholesterol reduction medication, and supplement my diet with over the counter fish oil (that I had been consuming as a bodybuilder for decades already) plus flax seed oil. I was also instructed to become more conscious of mentally monitoring episodes of accelerated heart palpitations, which given my devotion to high intensity gym workouts, and my obsession with biking fast and furiously around the neighborhood, I was able to realize that I push my 60 year old body to perform like I am a 30 year old. But it was comforting to learn that I need to advocate for myself with as much evidence and information possible when confronting the limited knowledge base of the Medical Industrial Complex.

This was game changer for my long-suffering post-disco anxiety disorder. But I still never know when I might experience another panic attack. I've read many contemporary books devoted to the subject, finding some too fraught with research details, too clinical for my layman's attention. The books I most relate to were memoirs of another anxiety sufferer, offering me hope sprinkled with entertaining anecdotes, inspiring me to write this book documenting my firsthand experience with this cautionary tale about abnormally altering your mind with an addictive drug of choice. It's comforting to know that palpitations can be truly miserable and disrupt the quality of life, but a frank discussion of the frustrations and progress in the science of addressing anxiety in the world we live in today, realizing that many of us were misdiagnosed as "major depressive", are finding solace in the suggestion that if we treat our palpitations as nothing more than a nuisance, cut yourself some slack with self-induced pressure (societal and physical), tweaking your lifestyle can strengthen your resistance to a life-sentence of panic attacks. And certainly, to any trauma inducing visits to the ER that by just writing about evoke an unsettling feeling that needs to be resolved.

CHAPTER 11
Treatment Advocacy

Since the 1950's, the science of addiction has focused its research on the neural basis of motivation and reinforcement behavior, publishing findings implicating a brain region, specifically a cluster of dopamine neurons, with reward-based learning. Drugs of abuse acquired since the beginning of mankind were later discovered to increase dopamine in the region of the brain associated with reward-based-learning, making them a part of our evolutionary process. Positive emotions such as euphoria and excitement were recognized as feelings chosen to be sought by our predecessors that influenced the behavior and physiology of an individual towards an increase in Darwinian fitness. At the same time, the pharmaceutical industry had begun furiously inventing, marketing, and profiting by bribing medical doctors to prescribe their newfound medicines with no regulation. Unfortunately, the research by scientists couldn't compete with the resources of the pharmaceutical giants in this country, failing to inform the public much less the government of the perils of unbridled long-term use of these legitimately prescribed and faithfully consumed prescriptive medicine. Ignoring the hazards exposed by empirical data provided by the scientific community, unregulated pharmaceutical medication freely dispensed by the medical community has caused a health crisis of substance abuse, addiction, overdoses, and suicides afflicting this country without any of the interference imposed on drug trafficking from outside our country's borders. Cocaine, heroin, and marijuana are no longer America's drugs of choice. It is prescriptive medication legally manufactured in the United States and distributed down the drug dealer chain from the commercial and sales representative promotion to the general public and licensed doctors' offices to the black market where the street dealer sells what the customer wants and becomes addicted to.

After 15 years of trying to repair the damage I inflicted on my brain's normal ability to release dopamine, which controls movement, emotion, perception, motivation and pleasure, I have come to the conclusion that the drugs I have ingested to heighten the feeling of pleasure to the point of euphoria has overstimulated my brain's normal reward pathways, making me incapable of being satisfied with "normal". My brain seems to always crave a heightened sense of pleasure, which is why I have a disposition to repetitious substance use and abuse. My adult life has chapters of addiction cycles alternating with periods dedicated to abstinence. Wash, rinse, and repeat. I was gifted with good cognitive skills, championing Darwin's theory that only the strong survive. But just as life is unpredictable, so is recovery, which requires constant vigilance to avoid relapse.

Fortunately, with the support of my understanding family, friends, my life partner Storm, and all the guardian angels (mortal beings and spiritual guardian angels) that see me, hear me, and boaster my confidence that I am "Okay", even on what feels like a bad day. My support system on this earth and the intimate conversations I have with those souls who have perished gives me the courage to persevere in my quest for nirvana.

Without bashing the current medical community, I have to give credit to the multitude of institutions dedicated to treating the mystery of substance abuse that I have committed to, listened to their advice, tried their prescribed treatments, and been able to professionally and graciously part ways when I feel like I am not making any progress, that I've reached a road block of my own design, and need to move on to another treatment option. I developed a proactive personality during my formulative childhood to make myself seen, heard and satisfied, and I believe that every human must advocate for themselves if they don't want to be treated like a herd of sheep, hindering their enlightenment with unresolved resentments and regrets. The medical community is employed by conventional human beings who have chosen to work in the healing profession by studying, training, and obtaining certification to practice their skills. But unfortunately, I find that a lot of these well-meaning health professionals are not only overwhelmed with the excessive inhuman caseloads they must maintain, but they are instructed to follow an addiction prevention model that was first discovered and employed 200 years ago, by Sigmund Freud, stigmatizing substance abuse as a disorder to society, relegating the health professional to a restricted litany of questions, preventing these health care providers from truly hearing, understanding, and ultimately helping each unique client they meet by taking the time to look away from their computer screen's form driven questionnaire that the client is required to answer, never really being seen much less heard beyond the limitations of the computer program's formula.

Not a fan of her craft or her celebrity manifestation, I give praise to film director Steve McQueen for casting novice actor Mariah Carey as a dowdy, tired, long-term social worker (no makeup!?!, and a trace of female upper lip facial hair !?!). Miss Carey's performance as a burnt-out employee of the Social Services Administration is spot on no reflecting the lack of empathy polluting the founding premise of this once benevolent government agency. As a physically and emotionally exhausted social worker, Miss Carey's apathetic character does not even bother to rise from her office chair to greet her latest client and challenge, "Precious". The brisk demeanor Miss Carey exhibited in this role is part of her character's defensive armor from the sad decline in the success rate and the loss of the original purpose of the Social Security Administration and local Social Service Agencies. But in this tragic but life affirming movie, the social worker's heart eventually melts like Scrooge when she begins to understand and empathize with Precious, her damaged and dangerously derailed client. I have encountered more suspicious and bitter health professionals who I will work with for a few months before requesting a change for another practitioner who I want to have some hope will make a difference in my well-being, physiologically as well as emotionally.

After reporting to the local Social Services offices shortly after my release from rehab in 2004, I found myself in the humble position of requesting food stamps and a monthly subsidy to contribute to my retired parents' household expenses. I had been gainfully employed since graduating from college in 1981, paying an ever-increasing percentage of my paycheck to taxes. I was not begging for a free handout. But the brief minutes of my assigned social worker's time coupled with the bureaucratic "red tape" paperwork required did not seem to grant me my pittance of a subsidy, regardless of my persistence. Two months later, I was approved by the more professionally organized Social Security Administration to receive handsome monthly benefit income based on the number of years and inflated salary I was paid and contributed to FICA, my nest egg to take care of me financially when I was no longer able to take care of myself. I filed a complaint with the board of appeals in Albany, New York for the lack of empathy and denial of a legitimate request for services with the local Social Services agency. Somebody has to have the gumption to advocate for themselves much less those that follow in this world.

There are guardian angels out there. I keep my confidence optimistic, believe in expelling good karma into the universe, stay humble, and take each day as it comes. But that doesn't mean that I take things for granted. Gratitude lists are the easiest trick to reversing the spin of some troublesome news. And nobody, not a lawyer, a case manager, a family member, a best friend or a TV commercial can fix problems better than advocating successfully for yourself. Do your homework. Keep records for reference. Set goals and revisit them. Share with anyone who will listen to you. Find a partner who is willing to pay attention to your histrionics, unconditionally love you without any reservations, and let you know that you don't have to always be perfect. That kind of healthy relationship will ensure you company through the otherwise depressing aging process. The price for fueling this drama-free home environment is to make amends when necessary, for your soul as much as for your partner's, and keep the focus on yourself; initiate changes in your own person, but don't expect or express dissatisfaction with your partner's short comings. Unconditional love is a humbling experience, and the synergy of a healthy relationship miraculously cures all.

Researching for books at the public library on the subject most imperative to this book and my personal welfare, I've discovered a plethora of published accounts documenting the fact that until the early 1980's, anxiety did not exist as diagnostic category. The leading diagnosis categorizing any mental disorder was "major depression", and the prescription of a multitude of nonstigmatizing anti-depressants was the status quo. Today, anxiety disorder is the most common form of officially classified mental illness, with respective medication, albeit physiological as well as psychological addictive due to their narcotically effective ingredients. As pervasive as this revelation is, the medical community, politicians concerned with the long-term effects of this treatment therapy, and new empirically proven research, the terrain of anxiety affliction that is so pervasive in the public's awareness via news stories of the new prescriptive drug epidemic and its consequences, is yet still misunderstood.

Every day, it seems the lead story on the local evening and national news programs involves prescriptive overdoses. If Michael Jackson and Prince (all born the same year of my birth, 1958, as well as self-sufficient Madonna) had been in contact, I would have done my best to try and save their victimized asses from the ill-intentioned support systems that did not preserve their lives but extinguished them. Now it's just me and Madonna. Lucky for me, I have excellent genes to make me look like I was born in 1980. Women don't get the respect to gracefully grow older like their male counterparts, embracing their silver hair, facial wrinkles that add character, and a decrease in their muscle mass index. Twenty-year-old vixens will target men 30 years their senior to satisfy an unresolved "daddy complex". Women, like Madonna, fall victim to media pressure to obsess about unnaturally maintaining a facade of youth and beauty. All the money that financially prosperous Madonna has continued to work for requires her to undergo the most contemporary non-invasive cosmetic surgery that I'm sorry to say has passed its shelf life and is now appearing frighteningly grotesque. The injections to her face have, like a person with an eating disorder or an addiction, elevated her treatment to the degree that her face is a distorted Halloween mask, filling the frame of a selfie shot like Kim Kardashian's buttocks.

Research into the history of humanity reveals its long-standing existence and treatment of anxiety, at once intimate and authoritative, and of the efforts to understand the condition from medical, cultural, philosophical, and first-hand experiential perspectives. Ranging from the earliest medical reports of Hippocrates (400 BC) to the later observations by great nineteenth-century scientists such as Charles Darwin and Sigmund Freud, they began to explore its sources and causes, to the latest research by neuroscientists and geneticists. Believing in science and not God, insight into the biological, cultural, and environmental factors that contribute to this afflict-tion has been my hope for the future and forgiveness for the past.

My story is just one unique experience of my struggle with anxiety, the myriad of emotional manifestations and anguish it can produce, plus the psy-chotherapists, medications, and other treatments (some outlandish, misdiag-nosed, blindly prescribed) to counteract the subject and condition of anxiety in today's world. As dark as some of the abnormal behavior I have detailed in this book, the crippling impact of high-anxiety and the handicap of relying on a narcotic substance to alleviate its discomfort, I am offering some alter-native activities and suggesting to advocate for yourself ways to manage and control it. You must believe you have the power to live with this condition, and someday hope to control it free of any other authority then your own.

Of all the status quo treatment options I have invested recovery time into, here is a list of some of my most highly beneficial and recommended exer-cises:

Hazelden 4th Step Inventory the Big Book refers to "the wreckage of your past . . ." in the wake of our substance abuse. Step 4 & 5 deal with how the past has affected our world within. When I first was left with the assign-ment of performing my virgin 4th step with nothing but AA literature to reference, I was lost and confused on how to satisfy my sponsor. I never completed the assignment, and soon after ended my allegiance to said spon-sor. Once I joined a more progressive, well read, open minded fellowship, I was introduced to the Hazelden 4th Step Inventory, from the revered Minnesota institute on recovery, Hazelden, hardly a heretic threat to the fundamentalist devotion to AA. The Hazelden approach avoids the blank page of an essay you want to ace but can't find the motivation to start. The 4th Step Inventory, available on the internet, is comprised of 155 questions, divided into three parts: 1. Childhood. 2. Adolescence. 3. Adulthood. The questions are psychologically organized to tap into the recesses of these three distinctly imperative periods of your life, encouraging you to respond intuitively rather than write what will impress your sponsor; there is no right or wrong answer. Some of the questions seem to repeat themselves, but there is an unspoken logic to this exercise. I was able to reveal secrets I thought I'd take to my grave and realized that a lot of my issues were not so important in the scheme of things.

I emphasis that being raised as the quintessential middle child had serious ramifications on my development, which the Hazelton 4th step helped me explore, and not take for granted. I believe that my disposition to experiment and ultimately suffer from drug addiction more so than my siblings could be explained by my motivation to get more attention from my parents, and the world; Darwin's theory of survival of the fittest. My use and abuse of substances has been classified as a reactionary behavior due to psychological and biological circumstances. I documented in my 4th step as well as in this book feelings of detachment from the family unit; the social inequality of feeling my brother and sister received more attention during my upbringing, which motivated me to achieve dominance and independence in my life choices during my adolescence and adulthood. Case in point: on the very first day I was emancipated from my parent's guardianship when I was transported to college, only to end up trolling the lawless streets of sex-saturated Times Square in 1976 at the age of 18 years old. How and why I ended up stripping and hustling could have been a risk my not so fully developed mind was receptive to engage in believing my parents would never find out, or care if I they did. It was my life, and I took control of it when I swore, I would never be dependent on my parents, or anyone, for financial, emotional, or spiritual support after fending for myself in the otherwise perfect middle class family of five I left with bitterness.

And the idea that the 155 questions that comprise the Hazelton 4th step are not gender, race, age, education, or sexual orientation specific makes it all the more universal. While I progressed with my 4th step, a particular horoscope column I would normally not give the time of day to printed these pearls of wisdom: "And with the realization of mortality regret tends to ripe, taking on an almost fantasy quality, as people remember their missed opportunities in one-dimensional, idealized way. For we tend to remember the past not as it was, but as we'd like to believe it was."

After completing and reviewing my 4th Step, I can now approach past events in a fresh perspective, so I can reanimate them. It's not a matter of reinventing my history but rather relocating its essence so I can experience it differently.

AA has over 80 years in the business of drawing alcoholics who don't have the financial or health insurance means to get a jump start on sobriety by spending 28 days at an inpatient rehabilitation center. But AA is not for everyone. What it excels in is a long track record, accountable for more meetings around the world in a day than the Pope holds mass. What it lacks is changing with the times. Its literature is outdated, and its model of abstinence is very limited: "Don't drink, go to meetings." Current research reasonably projects that about one of every 15 people who enter AA are able to become and stay sober.

SMART Recovery (Self-Management and Recovery Training) is an alternative to AA and its 12-step approach to recovery. Incorporated in 1992 as the Alcohol and Drug Abuse Self-Help Network, the international non-profit organization began operating under the name SMART in 1994. SMART differs from AA by not encouraging individuals to admit powerlessness over addictions, not using the concept of a "Higher Power", and not endorsing the disease theory of alcoholism The SMART approach is secular and scientifically based, and is intended to evolve as scientific research and knowledge becomes evidence for more progressive ideas on recovery. Addiction is - viewed by SMART as a dysfunctional habit rather than a disease, allowing that it is possible that certain people have a predisposition toward addictive behavior. There is less pressure in SMART meetings to be honest with the struggle to maintain a perfect record of abstinence, which is part of the recovery process if the stigma of talking about the relapse can become opportunities to learn and grow; each individual is encouraged to find his and her own path to their recovery. As opposed to the 12 steps, SMART recovery focuses on Rational Emotive Behavior Therapy (REBT) and other evidence-based cognitive-behavioral theories and techniques.

Cognitive Behavioral Therapy is a type of psychotherapeutic treatment that helps patients to pay attention to the internal dialogues we experience during the day, so that they may draw a link between these thoughts and the feelings, good and bad, they may invoke. Patients of CBT learn how to identify and change inaccurate thoughts that may reinforce destructive or disturbing thought patterns that have a negative influence on behavior and emotions. Giving credit to your cognitive skills empowers the patient that while they cannot control every aspect of the world around them, they can take control of how they interpret and deal with things in a practical manner.

Explore as many AA meetings to experience the different angle and vibe of the group conscience as well as the dedicated long-time attendees. Don't limit yourself to a meeting out of convenience. It's not a gym. It is a group meeting and an hour is a long time to clench your teeth and simmer resentments if the meeting is not your fit. The idea is to connect with other's in recovery. If AA meetings begin to seem tedious, organize a sober activity to interact in a non-competitive and manner, devoid of references to 12 steps. Sober Softball, Volleyball, Paintball, Bowling, ...

Journaling, especially in early recovery, is an excellent chance to start to break through the barrier of unconscionable thoughts privately, not exactly ready for public consumption. Writing about my personal experiences was a cathartic experience, never dreaming I could actually submit a query letter to publishing companies and literary agents to successfully attract the attention of the CEO of DonnaInk **Publications, L.L.C.** who took a chance publishing my subversive memoir of the debauched experiences I survived while educating as a cautionary tale. *Homo GoGo Man: A Fairytale About A Boy Who Grew Up In Discoland* shocked and impressed my family, acquired me consultation on investigative articles, museum exhibitions, and television shows interested in revisiting the now non-existent hedonism that made NYC the model that other international cities tried to emulate.

In the 21st century, euphoria is generally defined as a state of great happiness, well-being and excitement, which can be normal, or abnormal and inappropriate when associated with psychoactive drugs, manic states, or brain disease or injury. Stimulate the pleasure centers of the brain with social activities to generate a normal sensation of euphoria. Exercise is known to affect dopamine release producing euphoria through increased biosynthesis of endorphins. Listening, dancing, singing and creating music has the same effect as exercise. Copulation, either alone or with a partner, leading to an orgasm, is considered the pinnacle of human pleasure. Fasting has been associated with improved mood, well-being, and sometimes euphoria.

Recognizing potentially inflammatory people, places, and things, which can add fuel to the fire of unresolved and easily medicated emotions should be treated with a backup plan. Surviving any gathering of my immediate family, especially at the home of my origin, takes a lot of emotional restraint because the personality and property can allow me to slide back in time to behave like the confused adolescent who acted out for attention. Not very attractive as a 60-year-old with nieces and nephews to set a positive example of adult behavior. Gratefully, I have a BF, Storm, who can ground me. The Yin to my Yang.

Gratitude on days I don't feel well (mentally, physically, spiritually) is an easily accessible exercise, comparable to the power of prayer to those who believe. My BF Storm and my amazingly interactive exotic shorthair cat, Ford, are always at the top of my list. My family. Long-term friends. Good health. Establishing a bucket-list of wishes, desires, dreams and goals, and focusing on achieving at least one of them.

Facing the facts. Genetics, awareness to the complex changes in society. Acquiring and reading literature pertaining to this subject that is closest to my heart and hope that I can become more understanding of the issues involved in addiction.

Physical health has a direct correlation to mental health. Take care of your body. It is the vessel you will inhabit for 70, 80, 90, 100 years? See a Primary Care Physician, have tests performed that may preclude a potentially serious health condition besides a hangover, see a Dermatologist for superficial yet life threatening age spots, see a Dentist for X-rays as well as a good exam followed by a good cleaning to prevent dentures, and stand on the scale AT THE DOCTOR'S OFFICE to document your weight and height, to ensure that you are not evolving back into a prehistoric predecessor. As homo sapiens, we must avoid our own extinction.

The history of addiction. It's not just effecting your generation, or you for that matter. Stop personalizing your situation by volunteering for those who make you feel good about your life, someone else who could use your championing/mentoring, which makes you feel even better by someone appreciating you.

Love yourself.

Nirvana.

ABOUT THE AUTHOR

Christopher Duquette

I am beginning to field my title once more in NYC after a sabbatical in Rural New York to recalibrate from over technologicalization of my life; however, all things come full circle, and I missed the Big Apple. Currently, I hail in Jamaica Queens NYC and I am busily finding my path to the hidden niches of books, people, and readings . . . look for me throughout our great city and beyond in the 2017 - 2018 book-signing circuit.

If you have a venue, bookshop, store, grocery mart, location for a book reading and signing - I'm interested in hearing from you and so is my publisher, "Q" of DonnaInk Publications who delivers quality creations, heartfelt support, and authorial success.

Mostly, I want to say I appreciate you all as readers who have traversed the Disco Era or heard about it. If you are coming out, in the closest, straight and unafraid of life choices, or as gay as a blue-jay - thank you for being here and sharing this glimpse of history.

As a clean adult, post-era, I'm privileged to share a moment of history in recovery and pray the same for each of you.

~Christopher Duquette

2nd Spirit Books
601 McReynolds Street
Carthage, NC 28327

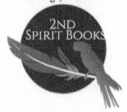

www.donnaink.com